MANAGE YO[
HEART ATTACK SURVIVOR

OVERCOMING ANGER, ANXIETY, AND DEPRESSION TO GET YOUR LIFE BACK AFTER TRAUMA

JON JOHNSTON

PRECARIOUSLY PERCHED PUBLISHING

CONTENTS

MY STORY

On August 21, 2015, I was sitting at a customer site with what I thought was a terrible case of heartburn. I had gulped down some Pepto-Bismol and chewed some antacid tablets earlier in the day, but it hadn't helped. I took off my glasses, laid them on the table in front of me, and rubbed my head in frustration.

Then I fell to the floor, dead from a widowmaker heart attack. My coworkers scrambled to figure out what was happening. They called 911, and when an ambulance arrived, the paramedics began CPR. A LUCAS device was placed on my chest. I was shocked five times on the way to the hospital with no response. I was shocked two more times in the emergency room at Hennepin County Medical Center in downtown Minneapolis, and my heart finally started beating on its own again. I had been dead for over twenty minutes.

A cardiologist placed a stent in my widowmaker artery, and I was put into a medically induced coma to save my brain function. The surgeon told my beautiful wife Heidi, "He is in God's hands now," as I was not expected to survive the night. Even if I did survive, the medical team cautioned that I wouldn't be myself anymore since my brain had been deprived of oxygen for so long. Heidi had to break the news to our three children. I have no idea how she found the strength to do that. I'm sure I would have become a blubbering, useless idiot if the roles had been reversed.

I remember nearly nothing about the ten days I spent in the hospital. For that matter, I remember very little about the rest of 2015. It took a couple of months before I discovered that many of my memories had either been blown to shreds or had disappeared completely. My cardiologist placed a second stent in January 2016. I continued to complain of debilitating headaches, and in June 2016, I was diagnosed with an anoxic brain injury.

Before my heart attack, I had never broken a bone or been admitted to a hospital. I tried to lead an active life. I was a Boy Scout leader for seventeen years, I coached youth soccer for a decade, and I have never smoked. Heidi is a very healthy person, so I wanted to stay healthy to keep up with her. Largely because of her influence, I have always eaten a reasonably healthy diet.

I never had any indications that my heart would have problems. I didn't have any of the big risk factors, and by all accounts, I'd been in good health. I spent months in denial that my heart attack was anything more than a scratch, but the truth is that part of my heart is dead because the major artery was blocked for so long. I was certain that my weakness and fatigue were problems I would easily overcome, just like I have everything else in my life. I spent a great deal of time and energy being angry and depressed, refusing to accept that I was limited in my physical abilities after my heart attack. I lashed out at my family, even though they had nothing to do with my pain.

For a while, I was apathetic. I didn't want to work, and there were days I fought myself just to get out of bed. I experienced headaches so severe I couldn't function; I'd lie awake all day in a dark room, unable to even look at my phone as the light caused unbearable pain. In my darkest moments, I wished I hadn't been saved.

It's been over six years since I died. I still work full-time as an IT consultant. In my spare time, I run a sports website, host a podcast, write, and shoot college sports photography when I get the chance. I try to stay active, both physically and mentally. Our family dog, Esther, requires a daily walk, so I try to walk two miles each day. I practice yoga to keep my strength up, although I'm not as diligent as I'd like to be.

I still wake up with a headache every day. I constantly fight fatigue. I have never stopped trying to improve my life so I can remain active, productive, and do the things I love. I have reclaimed most of my life and I know I've been fortunate.

The full story of my ordeal can be found in my memoir, *Been Dead, Never Been To Europe*.

What This Book Is Not

This book does not contain medical advice.

I am not a doctor or a healthcare professional. I work in IT, and no one would ever confuse me for a caregiver. It's not that I don't care, it's just that I'm not very good at it. That's why I work on machines.

If you have questions regarding a medication, condition, or treatment, please consult your doctor. If any information in this book contradicts direction you've received from your physician, please prioritize their guidance.

The details in this book are simply a reflection of my own experiences and are not meant to take the place of professional medical opinion.

What This Book Is

My goal is to inform other heart attack survivors about the steps I've taken to reclaim my life. I discuss the techniques that have worked for me. The vast majority of my days are free from anxiety or depression, I don't worry about the future, and I sleep better now than I ever have.

This book is broken into two sections: Struggles and Strategies. In the first section, I outline the struggles I have faced on my road to recovery. In the second section, I explain the specific strategies I have used to overcome those struggles. My hope is that this information will prove useful in your journey.

I have recovered my independence and optimism. I hope this book can help you do the same.

PART ONE
STRUGGLES

CHAPTER 1
ANXIETY

AFTER I CAME HOME FROM THE HOSPITAL, I PAID INCREDIBLY CLOSE attention to my heart. I felt every move my heart made. If I stilled myself, I could feel each beat. There were times I swore I could feel the blood moving through my arteries.

I experienced chest pains. This shouldn't have come as a shock since part of my heart had physically died because the blood flowing through my artery was blocked for so long. There was also a stent, a piece of mesh that had been placed to strengthen the artery and keep it from closing again. I had lived for fifty-four years without a stent; were the pains a sign of a problem, or was my body simply adjusting to this foreign substance? Is the stent metal? Does it matter? The stent is there to support the artery that had been weakened by my heart attack. What if the stent collapses? What if my body rejects it? What would I feel? How would I know? Would there be any warning, or would I just fall to the floor dead and not survive this time? Would I go to sleep one night and not wake up?

These are all questions I had when I began my recovery. I had a great deal of anxiousness around them. When you've been punched in the face by your own mortality, it's natural to have questions. There were no good answers, and without answers, my questions whipped themselves into anxiety.

I had to learn how to deal with the chest pains. It didn't take long to realize that I had to control my reaction to them. Others around me would notice each time I touched my hand to my chest or grimaced, and those closest to me—my wife, my friends, and my coworkers—reacted with abject fear. My heart attack had put them through great trauma, and I had no desire to subject them to more.

After I noticed their reactions, I stopped touching my hand to my chest and was more careful about the words I used to describe what I felt. They often asked about what was going on because they care about me and were frightened about what might happen next. They don't want me to die. I joked that they just didn't want to deal with the hassle of another heart attack. Humor was a way to ease the tension.

I learned not to use the term "chest pains," because that phrase would get me sent to the emergency room. Instead, I'd use words like "discomfort," only to discover that even that was a tad too strong. Finally, I learned to say that I felt a "twinge" so no one around me would freak out. Sometimes I'd call my chest pain a "quirk" or a "peculiarity." Although I downplayed the severity of these feelings to others, every tiny twinge in my heart was amplified in my mind because I was paying such close attention.

I wondered why my heart had betrayed me. It was as if my heart had become separate from me, something I could no longer trust. I wondered what I had done to make it angry. I'd led an active life, I tried to stay in decent shape, I never smoked, and I ate a healthy diet. Where had I gone wrong?

Eventually, I learned that I'd had a heart attack because my left anterior descending (LAD) artery was blocked by plaque from cholesterol. This didn't make any sense. I had never been told I had high cholesterol in my life.

I grew to believe that my heart had betrayed me on its own, though I still didn't know why. I thought that maybe if I paid close attention, I might catch it trying to betray me again.

I pretended that I was fine, but I was going quite mad inside. Anxiety felt like constantly trying to maintain my composure and not scream profanities at God or fall onto the floor in a fetal position. I was trying to hide who I really was, that I was afraid, and that I didn't understand what was happening because I really, really, *really* didn't want to go back to the hospital.

From talking to other survivors, I've learned that anxiety is incredibly common. It's understandable that a heart attack survivor would constantly worry whether they'll have another cardiac event. I don't remember my heart attack as well as others I've talked to remember theirs. They have recounted to me how much physical and emotional pain they experienced. They talked about how they were sure they were going to die, and how the physical pain was the worst thing they'd ever experienced.

The first time I heard about anxiety from someone else's perspective was when I spoke to a friend who explained that his brother-in-law had suffered a heart attack and was terrified of having another one that would kill him. I didn't understand his brother-in-law's reaction because his fear differed from mine. That man feared death. I have experienced death and no longer fear it. My greatest fear is surviving another heart attack but being nothing but a worthless blob. We both had anxiety about an unforeseen future.

Anxiety can be overwhelming, especially early in recovery. It can lead to lack of sleep, and sleep is crucial to the healing process, both physical and emotional. Anxiety brings its own set of problems. I couldn't sleep, and therefore, I couldn't function normally. I was stuck, unable to continue on with my life. Anxiety kept me prisoner. I know anxiety can manifest physically, and I frequently wondered if my pains were actually a result of mental anguish. The same applied to my nausea, dizziness, and elevated heart rate. I was determined to avoid another heart attack at all costs, but I was also desperate to stop going to the hospital unless it was absolutely necessary.

My anxiety attacks were the worst at night. I'd lie down to sleep, but then I'd start thinking about work, my relationships, or whatever was happening at the time. I'd think, *I need to go to sleep*, but thinking about going to sleep is a sure way to make yourself not go to sleep. I'd get frustrated, then I'd notice my heart rate was up, which made me more frustrated, angrier, and less able to sleep. I'd toss and turn, which

I knew would wake Heidi. Then I'd get upset at that possibility, leave the bedroom, go downstairs, and try to sleep on the couch. I would work myself into an explosion of anxiety, heart revved up like a super-charged engine. I would get so infuriated at myself that I would shake and pace.

The time ticked by slowly. Three o'clock would come and I would pray for three hours of sleep. At four o'clock, I told myself I would be fine with just two hours of sleep. By the time five o'clock hit, I'd plead for at least fifteen minutes of decent sleep. By the time I finally fell asleep at six or seven o'clock, it was time to get up and start my day.

This cycle did not make for productive days or good mental health. Thankfully, my

anxiety attacks became less frequent and less severe with time. They still occur occasionally, but now they don't overwhelm me or last terribly long.

It hasn't been easy to take control of my anxiety, but journaling and meditation have been helpful tools in the fight.

CHAPTER 2
DEPRESSION

Depression is a close relative of anxiety. They're not siblings, but more like first cousins. They might not always be seen together, but they're always sharing information. They tell each other about my weak points, what hurts the most, and what makes me feel inadequate. They operate as a tag team, one slapping the other gleefully as I lie down to sleep and think, "I wonder if I'll wake up in the morning?"

There's a difference between the two. I look at anxiety as a short-term mental state. It's the feeling of dread you get about something that may or may not happen, like waking up in the morning after a near-death experience. Anxiety is tactical.

Depression, on the other hand, is strategic. It's longer lasting. There's a level of ongoing sadness, and sometimes it moves deeper into a feeling of numbness where you feel nothing at all. These are not clinical, medical definitions. They are how I perceive the two: anxiety and depression.

Like anxiety, depression affects everything I do. It affects my motivation and my attitude toward the world. It causes fatigue, apathy, and poor sleep. I've never directly attributed my aches and pains to depression, but it wouldn't surprise me either. When I feel like nothing matters, my body responds in kind. My left arm stops giving a damn about moving all that well because my brain has told it, "Nothing matters, man. Why bother?"

I had an evaluation from a neuropsychiatrist after my brain injury diagnosis. The assessment included a questionnaire and a talk therapy session. He said the evaluation showed signs of depression, but I blew him off, insisting that I'd never been less depressed in my life. It wasn't a lie.

I have had thoughts of despair and suicide for most of my life; I've never lived on an even keel. It's always been up, down, and all around. My lowest points were remarkably brief, lasting only a few minutes. During those moments, my life became engulfed in darkness. I knew I had to hang on to life, that the voice in my head saying that "everyone would be better off without me" was temporary. Suicide is permanent. "Hanging on" is key to finding my way through the darkness. It feels very literal. In those painful moments, I hang on to everything that's good in my life, especially the people who love and care about me. The worst thing I could do would be to make them spend the rest of their lives asking, "Why?" or "What could I have done to prevent this?"

I have always told people that I would never own a handgun because I'd be most likely to use it on myself. I have zero doubt that I would have used it at some point; it would have been too easy. Quick, painless, and leave someone else to clean up the mess. Those periods of despair were an internal war between darkness and light.

I haven't reached those deep, dark depths of despair since my heart attack, but that doesn't mean I'm not depressed.

The "Why me?" question does come up periodically. It lingered in my mind quite a lot during my recovery, but not as frequently now that I've learned how to cope. I still don't have a good reason for why I had a heart attack. There's little history of heart disease in my family, and I didn't have many risk factors

. Why the hell did I have a heart attack, especially one so severe? I never saw it coming. If you'd asked me to make a list of the ways I thought I'd die, "heart attack" would have come after "being hit by lightning" or "being eaten by a shark."

The self-pitying questions ran through my head constantly. Why had God punished me? What had I done so wrong to deserve this? *Why?*

I thought about all the fun things I'd never do again.

I owned a twenty-foot fishing boat, an old tri-hull Alumacraft with a twenty-horsepower Mercury outboard motor on the back. It was fiberglass, so it was heavier than an aluminum boat. It was butt ugly, but it was perfect for fishing the lakes near my home in Minnesota. I will not say I loved that boat because it certainly wasn't exotic or luxurious, but I enjoyed the time I spent on it.

I had to sell the boat after my heart attack.

It just became too much to handle. Not only was it difficult to get in and out of the water, but the motor wouldn't start on the first or second pull and I was no longer capable of yanking on it twenty times to get it going. I had neither the strength nor the stamina. They don't make blue pills for outboard motors. It was the end of an era when I sold it, and I haven't been fishing much since. I still miss this great joy in my life.

My penis didn't work for at least a couple of months. Yanking on it didn't get it going either. The thought of not having sex again was worse than not going fishing! Thankfully, there's a blue pill for that problem, but I still wondered whether the act itself would kill me. Without fishing, a healthy sex life, and many of the other things I lost after my heart attack, I struggled to find meaning in the next phase of my life.

Heidi says I complained constantly about the things I could no longer do. I struggled with multitasking, which is required to do my job well. At work, I deal with many problems simultaneously, but after my heart attack, I couldn't multitask. I wasn't as quick to solve problems as I had been. I had always been the heroic savior of IT, coming up with quick solutions to complex problems, but after I died, I couldn't remember what I was working on from one moment to the next. I felt like a failure.

To make matters worse, I started drinking more. Alcohol is a depressant, so I was piling a depressant on top of depression, which did not help the situation. It momentarily helped me forget my situation, but sobering up meant I was right back where I had started, except I felt crappy on top of it all.

I had lost my identity. My cardiologist emphasized that I needed to have patience in my recovery. It was hard to figure out where my life was headed; I wondered where I'd be in five years when I was struggling to even make it through the next five minutes. It felt as though I was constantly asking, "Are we there yet?" like I was on a long road trip without knowing the destination. Day after day, month after month, it was the same struggle. Trying to figure out who I was and where I was going only accomplished the same thing as alcohol: piling depression upon depression.

I became angry with other people. I lashed out at them because of my circumstances when it was my own problem I couldn't deal with. I had to figure out how to get a handle on things. It got better over time, but the road was long and my progress was slow.

I still experience bouts of depression, but they aren't as severe as they were after my heart attack. Now, I accept that those periods are going to happen. The key is controlling them, not letting them control me.

CHAPTER 3
ANGER

Our emotions have a lot to do with how well we recover. Anxiety can cause a number of physical issues, including fatigue and high blood pressure. Depression can cause body aches and insomnia. Lack of sleep increases the amount of time it takes the body to recover. Websites and books on recovery all touch on these problems, but there often isn't much focus on anger.

Throughout my recovery, I've learned that anger is just as debilitating as anxiety or depression. Once you figure out how to deal with anxiety and depression, anger will still be there, dragging you down. It is deceptively dangerous because it sucks away your energy. It's almost as if you had a giant parasite attached to your body whose sole purpose is to drain you of life.

When I came home from the hospital, I was certain that my heart attack was nothing more than a speed bump and I would be back to my old self in no time. I was in complete denial. I felt that as long as I exercised and took the medicine my doctors prescribed, I would be as good as new. I had survived so many stupid moments in my life with little more than a scratch. Why should this be any different? Bad things happen to other people, not to me. I believed that I was more like Superman than most people; I knew I wasn't invincible, but I was damn close to it. By the time I turned fifty-four, I still hadn't broken a bone, had a serious illness, or been admitted to the hospital. I was sure I could talk my way out of hitting the ground during a fall from a thousand-foot cliff.

Reality hit in January 2016. I had experienced heartburn at a customer site, and although I tried to ignore it, I'd learned from my doctors and cardio rehab that ignoring problems with my heart would only make them worse. I called Heidi, who took me to the ER. That decision earned me another hospital stay and the placement of a second stent. The stent procedure went well, but my cardiologist had a big concern he wanted to address. Part of my heart was dead, he'd told me, limiting my recovery and my chances of ever returning to the life I led before my heart attack. He thought that I might eventually need to have a defibrillator implanted in my body to keep my heart beating correctly, but no matter what, there will never be a way to truly fix my broken heart.

This was the first time I fully understood the severity of my heart attack. I am not "normal." I will never be "normal" again, and there isn't a damn thing I can do about it. All I can do is make sure it doesn't get any worse.

I was overwhelmed with anger. I cried regularly. I was forced to face the fact that I had been lying to myself for months. I'd believed in a fantasy, that if I followed the doctor's orders, I could return to my previous life. I could feel like myself again.

I realized I was angry for two reasons. First, I had lied to myself. I couldn't understand this at the time, but I was going through the five stages of grief: denial, anger, bargaining, depression, and finally, acceptance. At the time, I believed that my problem was too complex to be boiled down to such a simple explanation.

But there I was, moving straight from denial into anger. Had I accepted my predicament earlier, I wouldn't have wasted months hoping for an outcome that was never going to happen. I could have charged right past the first stage of grief by opening my eyes to the reality of the situation. I had been told that part of my heart was dead, but I didn't accept it for months, only because I didn't believe it could happen to me.

The second reason I was angry was the unfairness and incomprehensibility of it all.

Why me?

There wasn't a single moment of my life that I had considered I might have a heart attack. I feared cancer after watching my father and grandmother die horrible, lingering deaths in the 1970s, but a heart attack had never been on my radar. I have never gotten over this. Six years later, the idea I had a fatal heart attack still seems unreal.

It's human nature to be angry after a life-altering event. We are forever changed. We are damaged and miss our previous selves, our former lives. It took me four years to write *Been Dead, Never Been To Europe*. I cried every time I wrote. I cried every time I edited. I've done podcast interviews, written website articles, and spoken with other heart attack survivors, and I've cried nearly every time I've told my story. I am unsure if this is undiagnosed PTSD or subconscious anger, but I lean toward the latter. Over the years, I've found ways to deal with my anger, but avoiding the subject certainly wasn't the solution.

The biggest problem with anger is the way it drains your energy. I never noticed this issue before my heart attack because I always had enough energy to make up for it. I didn't have to pay as close attention. When I focused on recovery, I noticed how quickly anger or frustration exhausts me.

It doesn't take much to see the debilitating effects of anger. You can perform an experiment:

Turn on the news. Browse social media. Recall a recent argument you had with someone close to you. Any of those actions will probably make you angry. Ruminate on whatever upsets you for a few minutes, and let it make you even angrier.

Notice the effects on your heart, brain, and body. (You get bonus life points if you don't get angry. Congratulations!)

Is your blood pressure higher? Did you give yourself a headache? Are you tired from the ordeal?

I end up with terrible headaches when I become frustrated or angry. In as little as ten minutes, I am too mentally exhausted to concentrate on difficult problems. I can feel the energy leave my body as if it were water running down a drain. Since I work on high-level IT systems, it's important that my mind is sharp and operating at top speed. I don't want to make a wrong decision that takes down systems or harms my customers' businesses.

The same concept applies at home. When I become angry or tired, I lash out at those around me. I become unpleasant (which is putting it nicely) and difficult to be around. My loved ones don't deserve this from me. They're the ones who have helped me recover, and they provide me with endless support. I'd rather maintain healthy, loving relationships with them than alienate them and be alone. They deserve better.

It took me a long time and a lot of hard work to figure out how to deal with my anger issues. Now, I make a diligent effort to keep a positive outlook, even when things are hard. Finding a new purpose for my life has helped me quiet most of the anger, and meditation and journaling have helped squash the rest. It's important to find a strategy that works for you and put it in practice before your life spirals out of control.

CHAPTER 4
MEMORY

SEVERAL MONTHS AFTER I WAS RELEASED FROM THE HOSPITAL, MY cardiologist asked me to meet with another heart attack survivor. I was excited for the opportunity because I felt that if I could help other people understand what they were going through, maybe it would help me too. The man I spoke with was a business owner, and he wanted to talk to somebody who was already down the road toward recovery. His heart attack hadn't been as severe as mine. He said he was working out at the gym and then woke up on the floor to a woman performing CPR on him. He was conscious when he arrived at the hospital and had only blacked out briefly.

My reaction to his story was complicated. I felt envious that his heart wasn't damaged severely, while mine was partially dead. However, I was grateful that I didn't remember my event, as I wondered how much more PTSD I would have suffered.

One thing we had in common was our struggles with short-term memory. He was accustomed to multitasking, being able to juggle several projects simultaneously. Not only did he have difficulty remembering what he was doing, but trying to keep everything in his head was also extremely exhausting. It was interesting to learn that he had memory problems after only blacking out for a short time. I have talked to several other survivors, and memory issues are a common theme in our conversations.

I assured him that his short-term memory problems would get better over time as mine had. I explained how bad mine had been when I first came home from the hospital, and hearing about our shared experience and my progress buoyed his spirits. He was a little discouraged to learn that I'd never fully recovered, but I reminded him that my event had been much more severe and that I was still working to reclaim my life.

I remember very little about the first several weeks at home after the hospital. Somehow I returned to work, although I was only able to work an hour or two a day before exhaustion overtook me. I passed a very complex certification, but I have no memory of even taking the test.

I have struggled to remember even the most basic of things, such as where I keep my underwear. They've been in the same drawer for twenty years. The same thing happened with the silverware in our kitchen.

Heidi would ask me to do something, and thirty seconds later, I would forget what it was. She might say, "Let's go out to dinner," and then a few moments later, I'd suggest we go out for dinner. At first, the people in my life would point out when things like this would happen, but they soon learned to let it go.

A few years later, Heidi and our kids admitted that my short-term memory problems were straining their patience. To keep from going crazy, they started playing games with me. They started assigning me chores, knowing I'd forget to do them. They'd all laugh when I walked away, knowing full well I'd be back in a minute to ask what I was supposed to be doing. I wasn't upset when they confessed because I knew I'd been driving Heidi crazy, asking her the same question throughout the day. Forgetting where I put my keys or wallet became part of my daily routine.

Underwear and silverware are important, but not nearly as important as remembering to take my medication at the proper time. Forgetting to take my pills has caused major problems. I often feared that I would die if I missed a dose. Heidi quickly learned not to trust me to take my medicine, so she kept it organized and made sure I took it. While I appreciated her help, I knew it caused extra work and worry for her.

One of my meds was prescribed to help my heart adjust to my brand new stent. I had no idea what would happen if I missed a dose. Was I supposed to take two to make up for it? Should I just forget about it? If I was scheduled to take a pill at eight o'clock, should I take it at noon or wait until the next morning?

Forgetting where I put my keys or my wallet was just part of a daily routine.

Long-Term Memory

Long-term memory was a different issue altogether. It took a couple of months before we realized how badly my long-term memory had been damaged. When my family would talk about a vacation we'd taken, I often wouldn't remember anything about it. I couldn't keep my kids' soccer teams and scout troops straight, even though I'd coached them and been their scout leader. It wasn't just hard to lose the memories; it hurt to realize I'd forgotten a lot of their childhoods.

I'd sometimes find myself at a customer site, working on a system that I had built, only to realize I remembered nothing about it. I've always kept documentation on the work I do, and it can be shocking to read through documents I'd written when I don't remember them.

Worse yet, people would walk up to me in a store and begin talking to me as if I were their best friend, but I wouldn't have a clue who they were. It was embarrassing. At first, I wasn't sure how to handle it. I often wore a hoodie as a disguise. If I saw someone unfamiliar approaching me, I'd walk the other way. If I were cornered, I'd tell them what happened and try to make light of the situation. I'd say, "I've been dead for a bit. It destroyed my memory. I have no recollection of who you are." The conversations weren't as awkward as I expected. People were surprised but didn't take offense. Most were understanding and kind.

Oddly, I forgot a lot of the books and movies I'd enjoyed, but not the music.

Growing up, I read every science fiction book I could get my hands on: Isaac Asimov, Ray Bradbury, Arthur C. Clarke, H. G. Wells, and Philip K. Dick. I know I read the *Foundation* series by Asimov, but I couldn't tell you a thing about those books now.

Despite the constant references to movies and television shows in our everyday lives, my memory of *Caddyshack*, *Happy Gilmore*, *Star Wars*, *Seinfeld*, and the rest are gone. I remember bits and pieces, but when people make these references, I have to just laugh and play along. I fake many moments in my life.

For some reason, music is different. It triggers something in me. I grew up with a mother who played music like other families watched TV. There was a stereo or radio playing in our house most hours of the day. Consequently, I remember the words to most old twangy country songs where the women were leaving and the cattle are dying, whether I want to or not.

The late 1970s and early '80s brought some of the greatest music in human history, in my opinion, at least. I haven't heard "Rat Trap" or "I Don't Like Mondays" by the Boomtown Rats in years, but I could sing them on request, word for word. I'm pretty sure no one wants that.

Memory of music brings me comfort. Old country music, like Hank Thompson, brings me right back to my childhood in western Nebraska, back to my mom. Sonic Youth, R.E.M., and The Replacements allow me to remember goofing off with my friends in college. Erasure and a certain cover of the Carpenters' "Top of The World" remind me of dancing with my children when they were young.

I discovered what I call "black holes" in my memory. There are many places I've been in my life that I no longer remember anything about. In April 2021, for example, I watched the University of Nebraska play Rutgers in a three-game series at Haymarket Park in Lincoln. It was the first time I'd been back to Haymarket since I'd been dead.

I've been to countless games at Haymarket over the years, both as a photographer and as a spectator, but I couldn't remember anything about it.

I remember sitting next to Noah, my oldest son, when a streaker ran across the outfield in a game against the University of Texas. Instead of covering his eyes, like a good father, I yelled, "Look at that guy!" We laughed as we watched the event staff try to chase him down.

I was there for another series against Texas when legendary Longhorn coach Augie Garrido was ejected from the game. Nebraska fans loved to hate Garrido, calling him "Soggy Burrito." As he walked out of the stadium that day, Nebraska fans narrated his footsteps: "LEFT, RIGHT, LEFT, RIGHT, LEFT, RIGHT!" Garrido paused mid-step and raised his head to taunt the crowd. Everyone burst into raucous laughter. Garrido was as magnificent a bastard as ever lived, which I say with the utmost respect. Despite a lifetime of memories from sporting events, these recollections are precious and few.

I used to know exactly where Haymarket Park is, but I could no longer find my way there. I pulled up the map on my phone, but it made little sense. That's why I call it a black hole: memories of what the park looked like had been destroyed, sucked into the void. They didn't even come rushing back when I walked through the gate again. It was a disturbing feeling, and for a bit, I felt sorry for myself. Luckily, when I met up with some friends and talked, it didn't take long to get comfortable. (For what it's worth, Rutgers swept Nebraska in that series, the first sweep at Haymarket since 2009, when my beloved Huskers were still in the Big 12. My friends blamed my presence for bringing ill fortune to Lincoln that weekend. Baseball fans are the most superstitious of any sport.)

My issues with memory have profoundly affected my ability to do my job. I am much slower than I used to be. IT requires constant learning, or at least it does for me, as most of my customers expect me to learn new technology quickly and teach it to them. It's much more difficult for me to learn now than it once was.

IT people are constantly dealing with IP addresses. When I am troubleshooting a problem, I have to remember the addresses of the computers I'm working on because problems frequently occur when the computers can't talk to each other. Before my heart attack, I could remember a stack of addresses with no problems. Now I can't remember a single one. I find myself writing them down or flipping back and forth between screens to make sure I have them correct.

My memory issues are severe because I was dead for so long; my brain was oxygen deprived for twenty minutes. In 2016, I was finally diagnosed with an anoxic brain injury. I worked with a neuropsychologist and a speech-language pathologist to understand my damage and make a plan to move forward with my life.

I've talked with other heart attack survivors who have not been diagnosed with brain injuries, and they still have memory issues. It seems to be a fairly common side effect. Any time the flow of blood to the brain is disrupted, damage is done.

I've accepted that I'll never recover the memories I've lost, the moments from my life that were sucked into the black hole. But with a positive attitude and the strategies I've developed to accommodate my poor memory, I am reclaiming my life.

CHAPTER 5
FATIGUE

IT SUCKS GETTING OLD, BUT IT DOES HAVE ITS BENEFITS. MY CHILDREN ARE far more interesting as adults than they were as children. I understand who I am and my place in the world more than I ever have. I'm not wealthy, but I worry less about money than I did before.

But then there's my body. When I was younger, I joked that I planned to use my body up by the time I died; I wanted to completely wear it out by living a full life. Now I regret making those jokes since I guess God took me seriously.

Fatigue remains one of my most frustrating problems, even six years after my heart attack. It is ever present.

I've always compared it to the Incredible Hulk walking into my bedroom every morning, carrying a refrigerator. On bad days, he lifts the refrigerator high over his head, then brings it down on me repeat-edly. He doesn't stop until my body has been crushed into pulp. He tells me to have a good day and then leaves the room. On these days, I do little but rest. I cannot. I am nothing but pulp.

On good days, the Hulk comes into my room and makes me get out of bed. He doesn't crush me into pulp with the refrigerator. Instead, he straps it to my back so I can carry it around all day. I do the best I can for the rest of the day, but there's a refrigerator strapped to my back.

When I tell others about my Incredible Hulk analogy, they say something like, "Yeah, that happens to me too." I think, *No, it doesn't, you condescending ass. You have no clue what this feels like. Even if the Incredible Hulk forced you to carry a refrigerator, it would be one of those little dorm refrigerators, not the Sub-Zero model I'm carrying.* Then I silently swear and fantasize about how I would kill them if it were legal. (Did I mention that I sometimes struggle with anger?)

Fatigue is persistent. It's inescapable. It's different from just being tired. It's the feeling that I just want to go to sleep all the time, all day, every day. No matter how much I sleep, it's never enough. I wake up still feeling groggy and exhausted. I have to fight my way through every day.

I never felt this way before my heart attack. I was a person who had boundless energy. I have spent the past six years blaming this problem on everything I can think of. I blamed my medication, and spent a long time trying different treatments. I even discontinued my medication altogether, after consulting my cardiologist, of course. I wanted to definitively see if any one of them was causing my fatigue. They were not.

I experience two types of fatigue: physical fatigue and neuro-fatigue. I'm careful to make the distinction because they are caused by two separate injuries, my damaged heart and a traumatic brain injury. Physical fatigue makes me exceptionally tired after exertion. A certain amount of this is normal and happens to everyone, but a major part of my body is permanently damaged. The heart must supply the rest of the body with oxygen in order to perform any physical activity, and my heart has to work harder than a normal person's heart to supply the same amount of oxygen. Naturally, it would be very difficult for me to have the same stamina as someone who hadn't experienced a heart attack and damaged their heart. I wish this weren't the case, but all the wishing in the world will never change reality.

I have spent the past six years working to understand fatigue. It's a particularly puzzling problem because before my heart attack, I rarely experienced any type of fatigue. I've been a high-energy person my entire life, always ready to keep going. I spent most of my life telling others that "tired" is just a state of mind, that you can simply tell yourself you're not tired and you won't be. That's how I lived my life. It's likely that I said this to someone who was dealing with the Incredible Hulk without understanding how they really felt.

Despite how quickly I get tired, I don't feel very limited by physical fatigue. I don't have a lot of physical strength; whatever I had was destroyed when I died, but I adapt by avoiding carrying refrigerators around like the Incredible Hulk. I don't attempt to lift heavy objects because I can't, and besides, my daily life doesn't require it of me.

I complete most of my activities without difficulty. I can mow my lawn without a problem as long as the temperature isn't over ninety degrees. If I push myself when it's too hot, I can become dizzy and need to take frequent breaks. I walk daily for exercise. I have completed many 5Ks, and I walk with Heidi in a 10K sponsored by the Big Ten every year. I'm worn out by the time I complete the 10K, but I suspect that's true for most people.

Every once in a while, I experience unexplained dizziness, which can be frustrating because I have to be careful about what I'm doing when it happens.

Mostly, I don't blame my physical fatigue for my inability to take part in activities,

but that has not always been the case. My family traveled to California in June 2016, nearly one year after my heart attack. Heidi and I went for quite a few walks on the beach, which was often frustrating for her because I couldn't walk as far as she wanted. One day, everyone went to Universal Studios without me. I decided to skip the trip because I didn't want to be a distraction or keep them from doing everything they wanted to do. Over the years, I've come to terms with my limitations, but I still work to build up my endurance when I can.

Mental fatigue is an entirely different matter. Traumatic brain injury survivors experience "neuro-fatigue," which is another way of saying that everything we do can be exhausting. Everything we experience is amplified. Stress is particularly tiresome. Before my heart attack, I ate stress like candy. I enjoyed the challenge presented by my job and never felt mentally exhausted.

•   •   •

For example, I have spent my long career repairing destroyed systems. In several cases, I assisted customers whose organizations had been infested with computer viruses. In one particularly bad case, a virus destroyed several servers, and I had to work twelve to sixteen hours a day for a couple of months to get the organization back in operation. The leadership of the company was furious because they lost data and the use of their systems. I was frequently yelled at, but it didn't bother me because I knew they were not upset with me personally.

I enjoyed being the hero, putting my skills to work to solve a complex, important problem. Even though customers expressed their frustration, they were always happy I was there in the end. Fatigue did not get in the way of performing my job expertly.

Now, only a short period of stress can entirely exhaust me and render me nonfunctional.

Recently, I received a message early in the morning that there was a problem with one of my customer's servers and people were complaining. The customer asked if I had made any changes or if the system had been hacked. I became very upset at the possibility that I'd done something wrong. When I returned the call, I discovered that only one person had complained, the server hadn't been hacked, and I only needed to make a few slight adjustments to satisfy the complainer. The entire process lasted no more than twenty minutes.

In that short time, I went from having a slight headache to a debilitating headache. The pain was so severe that I couldn't even bear to look at the light from my computer monitors. I tried to calm myself down, but that short period of stress left me nonfunctional for the rest of the day. I did nothing but lay in bed and wait for the day to finally end. It was extremely frustrating, but I knew that if I tried to push myself harder, I would only make things worse for the next day.

I've tried to determine whether there are specific areas of my life that exhaust me more than others. Physical overexertion can cause headaches, so I am very careful about what I do physically. Every once in a while, I want to feel manly, so I pick up something heavy, like a box full of books. Inevitably, I pay the price: an instant headache and dizziness. I often have to remind myself that I'm not the Incredible Hulk.

I have discovered several specific tasks that exhaust me mentally.

I can't do math anymore. I can do simple addition and subtraction, but I used to understand advanced math well enough to enjoy sports analytics. I could easily understand graphs and scatter plots about my favorite football team, the economy, or whatever subject was presented. Now, trying to make sense of a scatter plot can leave me nonfunctional. I have to avoid math.

Anything that involves a lot of variables exhausts me quickly. I am frequently called upon to work on firewalls and database systems, both of which require me to hold many variables in my head. Trying to remember the various pieces that comprise a database system is exhausting. It's so disheartening to feel drained by the work I love so dearly.

Another common problem I have is dealing with human speech. As we grow older, it's hard for us to understand speech when there is a lot of background noise. During the pandemic, my family got together for meals or to watch football games. These gatherings often included multiple people in the same room, all talking at once while the TV was on in the background. It shouldn't have been a surprise that I found myself overwhelmed with a headache, which then caused me to be cranky. I was frustrated with my limitations and said things I didn't mean. I often had to remove myself from the situation until I could regain my composure and replenish my energy.

I do everything I can to avoid noisy restaurants. Several times, I've walked into a restaurant for dinner and am struck by a wall of sound. In those cases, I just turn around and walk back out again. I know what's in store for me if I chose to eat there: I wouldn't be able to hear the waitstaff or the conversations of the people at the table. I'll end up cupping my hand over my ear in attempt to block out background sounds. The other members of my party will either become frustrated with me or stop talking to me altogether.

When I leave, I will be exhausted.

I've struggled with many physical and mental challenges since my heart attack, but fatigue has been the hardest to manage. It impacts my everyday life, my work, and my relationships in a way that is difficult to avoid.

CHAPTER 6
SLEEP

I'VE HAD PROBLEMS WITH SLEEP FOR MOST OF MY LIFE, BUT I DISMISSED them by telling myself that I just didn't need as much as other people. I survived on four or five hours of sleep a night. I convinced myself that sleep was for the weak. During all the hours other people spent sleeping, I was working. I told myself that I was getting ahead of them, that I'd live eighty years by the time I was forty. A fat lot of good it did me.

When I lay down to sleep, my mind came alive with a fury, worrying about tomorrow's work, ideas I'd like to write about, or things I wish I hadn't said twenty years ago.

I'd contemplate the mundane: is a hot dog a sandwich?

I'd solve world peace, world hunger, and invent faster-than-light-speed space travel. I wrote entire novels in my head. I tossed and turned all night, then finally fell asleep thirty minutes before it was time to start another day. Sadly, I always forgot the genius ideas I'd come up with during the night.

There were a few times that I slept so little I began to hallucinate. Once, I saw a small dog running around at my feet while I was driving home from a customer's site. Another time, I was driving home on autopilot and freaked out, thinking I was in Seattle despite being north of Minneapolis.

It was not a healthy way to live.

It never occurred to me that I'd have been better off if I learned to quiet my mind. I thought that this was how successful people thrived: welcome stress as a challenge, not an obstacle, drive yourself to the edge of consciousness, and make sure you're more productive than everyone else.

I accepted my poor sleep as a way of life, the price I paid for success. In hindsight, it was an incredibly foolish way to live. The extent to which it hurt my creativity and decision-making is anyone's guess.

Lack of sleep is especially harmful after trauma. If I don't have a good night's sleep, my chances of having a "Hulk Smash" kind of day go through the roof. I wake up with a worse headache than if I'd slept well. Aches and pains are amplified. Apathy is increased. Motivation is lacking. It's incredibly difficult to get up and going in the morning.

After I was diagnosed with a traumatic brain injury, part of my recovery involved therapy with a speech-language pathologist (SLP). During therapy, the SLP informed me that the brain repairs itself during deep sleep. She talked about how sleep gets rid of all the "tangles" in our brain. I'm no neurologist, but it seems comparable to an automated procedure that clears out the clogs from the plumbing in our brains. If you don't sleep well, the clogs don't get cleared and your chances of having brain fog are much higher. Some researchers have found that those who don't sleep well in middle age have a greater risk of dementia, something I imagine everyone else finds as terrifying as I do.

The world is a much better place when I've had a good night's sleep. I am much better able to handle stress. I can focus more clearly, which means I can handle the complex problems my job requires. I am less agitated and better to the people around me.

I have not completely solved my sleep problem. My goal is seven hours of sleep a night, but I rarely meet it. I routinely wake up after four or five hours, knowing I need to sleep more. I can often put myself back to sleep to get an extra two or three hours, but I would prefer to have uninterrupted sleep. If I can't fall back to sleep, I prioritize taking a couple of naps during the day.

My schedule is very different now than it was before my heart attack. Before, it wasn't uncommon for customers or friends to receive emails from me at two or three o'clock in the morning. Now I'm in bed at eleven thirty and typically get up at six o'clock. I have experimented with moving the times around to obtain my goal of seven hours, but I'm more consistent if I set a target bedtime.

The good news is that I can fall sleep almost instantly, which I'd never been capable of doing before, because I have taught myself to quiet my mind before bed. It's rare that I lie down with the anxiety of thinking I might not wake up in the morning. Even when I do, I can dismiss it without it taking over my life and making me miserable.

What is most interesting is my attitude toward other people's sleep habits. I used to consider the people who liked sleeping to be lazy because I thought they had a poor work ethic, but now I admire them. I want to be more like them.

Part of my problem is that my body is unwilling to change.

It's more than just setting a new habit. It's as if my body is saying, "You refused to sleep for your entire life and now you want to change all that? We are going to fight you tooth and nail." I am convinced that there is a small faction of anti-sleep protesters in my brain who refuse to accept this new change.

PART TWO
STRATEGIES

CHAPTER 7
CARDIO REHAB

WHEN I GOT HOME FROM THE HOSPITAL, CARDIO REHAB WAS THE FIRST outpatient program I attended. I went to a nearby clinic for an hour-long group session three times a week . We attached our heart monitors and completed a light warm-up before spending ten minutes each on a stationary bike, a treadmill, and a stair stepper. The nurses in charge monitored our heart rates, asking us about our stress and exertion levels. A metronome guided the rhythm and set the pace.

The exercise was followed by a fifteen-minute educational session in which we learned about the heart, proper diet, reading food labels,
and maintaining our overall health.

I attended cardio rehab without arguing because I was told it would improve the strength of my heart. I never felt strained by any of the exercises, and in fact, I was frequently told to slow down and not push myself too hard. *cardio rehab*

Several very important benefits came out of my time in cardio rehab: I learned my limitations, I grew to understand how important it was to pay attention to potential problems, and I gained confidence.

Limitations

Even though I didn't want to admit it, there are limitations on what I can do. The best way to predict whether an activity is appropriate for me is to understand its METs score. The METs test measures the amount of energy it takes to perform a physical activity. If a cardiac patient knows their METs score, they can choose activities that are suitable for their ability level. For example, moderate activity, ranked from 3.1 to 6.0, includes:

- Walking a dog
- Carrying a fifteen-pound load upstairs
- Gardening
- Vacuuming
- Walking 3.4 miles per hour on a level surface
- Doubles tennis
- Vigorous activity, ranked greater than 6.0, includes:
- Swimming
- Soccer
- Push-ups or sit-ups
- Jogging/running
- Shoveling snow by hand
- Carrying a thirty- to sixty-pound load

When I arrived at cardio rehab, my METs score was 2.4. Gardening was off the table, and jogging was out of the question. At least I didn't have to help with the vacuuming. By the time I graduated, I measured 4.3. My list of approved activities expanded.

Do I follow the METs recommendations religiously? No.

I have taken part in 5K and 10K walks. I bought the last brand new mountain bike left on earth during the pandemic and spent the summer of 2020 biking all over town. There were times that my heart rate went as high as 180 beats per minute and stayed there for a while. When I asked my cardiologist about such a high level of activity, he reminded me that my target rate was around 145. It was okay for my heart to reach 180, but I risked arrhythmia if it stayed too high for too long. Riding twenty-five miles was okay. Riding one hundred miles was not. It gave my ego an enormous boost for him to even consider I could ride one hundred miles in a day.

What good is the METs score if I don't follow it?

Well, it certainly gets me out of vigorous activities I don't want to do. I have shoveled very little snow since my heart attack. I don't carry large printers around anymore. The guidelines give me a clearer idea of what I'm capable of and what I should stay away from.

Understanding your METs score and your limitations will help you avoid overexertion and additional damage to your heart. By getting regular, appropriate exercise, you can slowly work to improve your score and strengthen your heart muscle.

Don't Ignore a Potential Problem

I realized how detrimental it is to ignore the signals your body is sending. The educational sessions at cardio rehab helped me understand that it's critical to listen to your body. If you think you're having another heart problem and ignore it, you can do serious damage to your heart.

I don't want to lose the progress I've made on strengthening my heart. I don't want the life I've worked hard to reclaim to be lost just because I'm too stubborn to go to the ER or talk to my doctors about how I'm feeling. Ignorance is not bliss. Ignorance is very foolish.

Sometime after my heart attack, I had a frank conversation with a family friend. He confessed that he got chest pains after bicycling for ten miles and asked me what he should do about it. I told him he needed to be checked out by a doctor because physical pain from exercise is not a good sign. He didn't want to see his doctor. He used the "ignorance is bliss" line, then said, "Maybe it'll get bad enough to kill me. I'd be done. That wouldn't be so bad."

"That's the problem," I said. "It won't kill you, it'll just destroy you. They're not going to just let you die. That's not what they do. You'll end up living in a wheelchair with an oxygen tank. Is that what you want?"

During cardio rehab, I realized that they're not going to let you die even if that's what you want. It is the job of paramedics and EMTs to save your life. If I had another heart attack, chances are good that I would be saved. But at what cost? I would end up with more damage than I currently have and a life that is less independent, less fulfilling, and less joyful.

Confidence

It took me a couple of years to realize how much confidence I gained from cardio rehab. It helped me believe that my heart, my traitorous heart that betrayed and killed me, wouldn't do it again.

This was an extremely important lesson to learn. I hate going to the hospital. I made mistakes early in my recovery that caused avoidable trips to the ER.

I had to walk a fine line; I had to learn how to recognize when my chest pains were the sign of a problem, but balance that with my desire to stay out of the ER.

It took a long time. Six years later, I still haven't entirely arrived at a happy medium. I'm not sure I ever will, but I don't get anxiety about it anymore. My decision to go to the doctor isn't driven by fear, but analysis. It's made life more livable.

CHAPTER 8
PHYSICAL EXERCISE

I CANNOT FIX MY HEART. IT WILL NEVER BE WHOLE AGAIN. IT WILL NEVER be as healthy as it was before my heart attack. I cannot fix my brain. I can't go back.

What I can do is try to prevent my health from getting any worse. Exercise is a crucial component of maintaining my health, and the best way I've found to stay active is to walk every day.

There are wonderful trails all throughout my suburban neighborhood in Minnesota. I can walk out my back door, get on a trail, and walk for many miles, far more than I can safely walk.

Winter can be tough, so we have a treadmill at home. Walking on the treadmill isn't my favorite thing, but it's better than nothing. I usually listen to music while I'm on the treadmill, and if I'm walking outdoors, I listen to music or a podcast.

Walking doesn't just help me stay physically healthy, it helps my mental health too. A long walk can clear my head of the problems from that day. If I get stuck on a tricky issue at work or have a conflict with someone in my life, I can go for a walk to sort it out, often out loud. I don't care if other people can hear me or if I look like a crazy person, as I frequently wave my arms while I'm talking.

When I travel, I still make an effort to walk, even if there aren't trails nearby. Without that daily exercise, my body gets stiff and I become cranky. Exercise also helps me have productive sleep.

Unfortunately, walking doesn't do as much good for my upper body strength as I'd like, so

I practice simple yoga. I've been out of practice with yoga lately and need to get back to it. It does wonders to build muscle and clear my head. Planking and push-ups are other great ways to focus on the upper body, if your body can handle the exertion.

In December 2021, I was working for a customer in Dallas, Texas, and they invited me to their Christmas party at a virtual reality center. There were about twenty of us. We broke up into teams of four. When it was my turn, our team put on backpacks, virtual reality headsets, and headphones. We were handed a device that resembled a gun. When the game started, the headset displayed a simulated environment. We walked around a platform, shooting at members of the other team and trying to complete objectives. It was very similar to Capture the Flag.

I was apprehensive about trying virtual reality. I worried it would mess with my brain because of my brain injury, and I was sure I'd get a severe headache or mess up my balance. Something terrible was bound to happen, and I just knew I would end up trying to recover for a day or two in bed.

My desire to play and my fascination with virtual reality eventually overrode my fear.

The game lasted twenty minutes, and when we removed our gear, I was covered in sweat. I was exhausted, which surprised me. I was even more surprised to discover I wasn't the only one. Even younger, physically fit guys were dripping with sweat and talking about how exhausting it was. One of my teammates mentioned that

he had a virtual reality headset at home and enjoyed playing games with his son. I learned that VR games came in a variety of levels of intensity. It's important for anyone, but especially cardiac patients, to start with easy games before attempting virtual roller coaster rides or learning how to fly.

Because of my experience at the party, I bought two virtual reality headsets for Christmas. I purchased several games, including Beat Saber, the game advertised on commercials where players swing at blocks that are flying at them. VR offers a great mix of exercise, fun, and escape.

It didn't take long to discover Supernatural, a fitness application

that includes several types of sessions: Flow, Boxing, Meditation, and Stretching. There are high, medium, and low intensity choices, and the workouts last anywhere from seven minutes to one hour. The sessions are set to a variety of music, and coaches assist you through the process. I enjoy boxing the most, but I can't do the high-intensity workouts because my heart rate gets too high. During the medium workouts, my heart rate generally stays in the 150–170 range, and I stick with workouts that are no longer than fifteen minutes to avoid keeping my heart rate elevated for too long.

Virtual reality is yet another experiment I'm trying. It takes time to find the right combination of appropriately challenging exercises with something that maintains your interest. Still, I have to force myself to exercise. I've forced myself to do the Supernatural workouts when I was feeling tired, particularly from mental fatigue. I know chemicals are released in the brain during exercise that can improve your mood and mental clarity. I don't care. I track how I feel before and after workouts in a journal, and I've discovered that the workouts are reju-venating, much like meditation. My headaches lessen in intensity. I get physically tired from the workouts, but I feel much better. Even though I know all of this, I still have to force myself to exercise every time. I know it's good for me, even if I don't want to do it.

I track my heart rate with my Apple watch. There are many options for fitness trackers on the market, and they all have heart monitors. I've used a Fitbit in the past, which I liked, but the Apple watch pairs nicely with my iPhone and makes it easier to track my sleep, access my calendar, or use a journaling app.

Although I track my heart rate, I never take my blood pressure.

The only time my blood pressure is taken is when I'm at a doctor's office. I don't even own a blood pressure monitor. It would only drive me crazy.

For example, I often get

slightly dizzy when I stand up too fast. If I owned one of those blood pressure monitors, I would use it during a dizzy spell to ensure it's not a pressure issue. I am the curious type, after all. What happens if

I think it's off? What happens if it's not what it should be or what I expect? I know myself well enough to know that the scene would play out like this:

I think there's something wrong. I get anxious.

I take it again.

It's higher because I'm anxious.

There's something wrong.

I take it again.

It's still higher.

I take it again.

(Lather, rinse, repeat.)

Taking my own blood pressure would result in a feedback loop from hell, or a ticket to the ER, which is the same place. I don't want to go to the ER unless it's an actual emergency. A blood pressure monitor would only cause anxiety, which I don't need.

Besides, I've already made too many trips only to find out there was nothing wrong.

After one false alarm, my cardiologist gave me some helpful advice. He said that if I felt that there was a problem with my heart, I should elevate my heart rate by doing something strenuous. Run around the block. Run up and down the stairs. If there is really a problem, the pain in my heart will increase. This is one reason I track my heart rate.

I've taken his advice many times, and I've never needed to make another trip to the emergency room. That simple bit of wisdom has helped me gain more confidence in my physical well-being and my ability to identify a real problem.

When I asked my cardiologist whether I should take my blood pressure periodically, his answer surprised me: taking your blood pressure more than once a week is a waste of time because it doesn't change much. If you have questions about measuring your own blood pressure, consult with your physician.

It's tough to find the will and energy to exercise. It's a constant battle, especially when I'm tired. I know that going for a two-mile walk will rejuvenate me, but I still have to force myself to do it. I start to feel terrible if I don't exercise regularly. I am lethargic, listless, and low-spirited. I am groggier than I would be otherwise.

One of my biggest goals is to improve my physical fitness. Since I've already been dead, I have every excuse available to let myself go, to turn into a blob. But there's still so much left in the world that I haven't seen. I hear Hawaii is beautiful, and I've still never been to Europe. I will not get to visit those places if I'm in a motorized wheel-chair with an oxygen tank strapped to the back. I plan to do as much as possible with the rest of my life.

If I can stay active until late in life, perhaps I can make fun of my adult, middle-aged children when they let themselves go.

Be sure to speak to your cardiologist before you begin an exercise regimen. It's important to understand what your heart can handle so you can develop an appropriate exercise plan that won't put you back in the hospital from overexertion.

CHAPTER 9
DIET

THIS CHAPTER ISN'T ABOUT SPECIFIC DIET RECOMMENDATIONS. THERE ARE countless books, websites, and other resources out there about the best foods for cardiac patients. Instead, this chapter is about my experiences with food after my heart attack.

I had never considered my diet to be unhealthy. Heidi stays in very good shape, and a big part of that includes how we eat. I've always been determined to stay active so I can keep up with her, so my diet mirrors Heidi's. We never ate a lot of meat, especially beef, and we try to maintain a balanced diet that includes a lot of fruit and vegetables. I don't drink very many soft drinks. I am terrified (no exaggeration) of energy drinks, since I'm not sure what they'd do to me, so I avoid them.

Salt

One change we made after cardio rehab was to eliminate salt. We went through the food we ate regularly to identify the ingredients or meals that had a high sodium content, and then we eliminated it from our diet. This included a lot of canned soups. They're easy to make, great when it's cold, but they are loaded with sodium.

The downside to eliminating salt was that everything tasted awful. The meals we cooked at home were so bland because they didn't contain the salt my taste buds were accustomed to having. Over a few weeks, my taste buds adjusted to the new no-salt diet. Once we got used to it, whenever we ate out, everything tasted like salt. Everything. It didn't matter if it was fast food or dinner from an upscale restaurant. Enjoying food was difficult.

It became such a problem that I brought it up at one of my cardiologist appointments. He insisted that I didn't need to worry about my salt intake as much as some other heart patients. It turned out that I didn't need to cut salt completely from my diet, but he did want me to follow regular dietary guidelines and make sure that I wasn't eating food with a high sodium content. I was relieved to add salt back to my food.

If you're wondering about your diet, ask your doctor. Your cardiologist will tell you if you need to switch to a low-salt diet. It's important to be your own advocate and ask questions.

I don't eat a lot of fast food. It's just not enjoyable to me. Every once in a while, I'll get a craving for a Whopper or a Big Mac, so I'll stop by whatever fast food chain is close to my job site. I rarely enjoy it. It never tastes as good as I imagined it would, and ten minutes after I've eaten, I feel like a ten-pound rock is in my stomach.

We prefer making our own food at home. During the warmer months, I smoke a lot of meat, such as ribs or chicken, but very little beef. I have created my own rubs that are low in salt or salt-free. During the winter months, I make many of the soups I enjoyed before my heart attack, and I just adjust the recipe to include less salt.

There are plenty of spices and herbs you can add to your food to replace or reduce your reliance on salt. Mrs. Dash is a brand of seasoning commonly used to provide flavor without salt, and they offer a wide variety of mixes that are all very good. Marshalls Creek Spices is another of my favorite brands that offers great seasoning mixes, including many choices without salt.

Salt is cheap and abundant, so it's easy for manufacturers to include it in their seasoning mixes and rubs. When I find a new mix, I'm always eager to look at the ingredients. More often than not, salt is the first ingredient on the list. It's a cheap way to make everything taste better, but too much sodium can lead to high blood pressure and heart disease, making it particularly dangerous for most cardiac patients.

I read food labels more now than I ever did before. I am shocked, SHOCKED, at the amount of sodium, sugar, and fat used in processed foods. I always suspected that this was the case, but it's astounding when you really start paying attention to it. Now, whenever I'm going to purchase a new rub or seasoning mix, I always check the nutrition label. I check every different soup I purchase. I made the mistake of checking ramen noodles once, and I was appalled at the sodium content and quickly put that packet of death back on the shelf. I am especially wary of soup mixes that bill themselves as healthy.

Being more cognizant of what I purchase at the grocery store has changed how I view food. I am much more likely to cook my own soups than I was before. I have found pleasure in creating my own rubs to use when I smoke chicken or pork ribs.

If I eat something that's high in sodium, I try to make up for it by not piling on through the rest of the day. If I eat fast food for lunch, I don't eat out again for dinner.

I especially enjoy going to Super Target, finding a product infused with sodium, and showing it to other shoppers. They frequently scurry away, terrified, but only rarely do they call security. I feel that it's necessary to spread the message about sodium. Perhaps I should start going door to door.

Fat

I learned a lot about the different types of fat in cardio rehab. There are four types: saturated, polyunsaturated, monounsaturated, and trans fats. Saturated and trans fats are bad for your health. Unsaturated fats are healthier.

Saturated fats include foods like pork, fatty beef, poultry with skin, cheese, butter, lard, and cream. Trans fats include fried foods, commercially baked goods, such as cakes or cookies, nondairy creamer, and microwave popcorn. Unsaturated fats come from plants, fish, nuts, seeds, and oils that are liquid at room temperature, such as olive or vegetable oil.

Basically, watch the salt and watch the fat. Eat fish twice a week instead of red meat. Check the labels on everything you buy at the store.

So much for mixing up the bucket of lard and salt I used to snack on during football games. Maybe it's for the best.

I enjoy everything in moderation. Every once in a while, I'll have a steak. I'll eat fast food, then regret it later. I don't worry that cheating occasionally on an otherwise healthy diet is going to kill me. I enjoy fruits and vegetables more than ever. Throw in some nuts for a snack and I'm okay.

The one thing I'm still working on is sugar. I have a big sweet tooth. Dark chocolate might be the best reason human beings evolved. I know I could drop ten pounds in a snap by completely cutting unnecessary sugar out of my diet. I've done it before. I'm sure I'd feel better, but I'd have to give up cookies, ice cream, coffee creamer, cake, candies, and most non-water-based drinks. I'm not sure that a life without chocolate is a life worth living.

Alcohol

I was a heavy drinker for most of my life. I quit drinking for good in April 2020. At the time, I was taking a brain seizure medicine called Divalproex. I was also drinking a lot of alcohol. Mixing the two was a stupid thing to do. Divalproex can be used as a mood stabilizer, and it's frequently prescribed to people with epilepsy to control seizures. In my case, it was to treat my severe headaches. By taking both alcohol and Divalproex, I was mixing two depressants together, then wondering why my life was terrible. I was drinking a lot of alcohol to help with the headache pain from my brain injury. If I drank enough, I felt nothing. The pain would be gone for a short while, which was what I was looking for, but I woke up the next morning feeling horrible. I'd start drinking again to get rid of the pain.

I knew the cycle would eventually destroy me. It was destroying my relationship with my friends and family, particularly my wife, and it was only a matter of time before I destroyed my career, my marriage, and the rest of my life. I had to choose between alcohol and life, and I chose life. I've had no alcohol since, and I have zero cravings for it.

I have many things I still want to do with my life. I want to become a successful author, travel with my wife, and continue to be a successful IT consultant until I retire from that career and start another. I don't want to be a drunk. Heidi deserves better. My children deserve better. My friends and customers deserve better. Even I deserve better.

Several of my doctors have suggested that my alcohol consumption contributed to my heart attack. I dismissed this idea every time it came up. It was much easier to blame genetics. The problem with alcohol consumption isn't the beer or wine itself, but how you let it take over your life. When you're drinking too much, you stop doing whatever else is necessary to stay healthy. You stop exercising. You stop eating well. You turn into a blob.

When people ask me what it's like to not drink anymore, I tell them it's like being freed from prison. I still struggle with pain every day, but I go forward with a clear mind and a healthier body. I feel better. I am much more productive. I am no longer destroying my relationships.

It's a good place to be.

CHAPTER 10
MEDITATION AND
MINDFULNESS

I USED TO ROLL MY EYES WHEN I HEARD PEOPLE TALK ABOUT MEDITATION.
I'd get a mental image of a Buddhist monk meditating in a cave or a
hippie sitting in Lotus position, legs crossed, hands resting on their
knees, fingers together. All I could think was, "What a poser."

Meditation wasn't for me. It was for people who had time to squan-
der. I was going places and doing things, not sitting around wasting
my time thinking about my place in the universe. I wasn't trying to
"find myself." I was well aware of who I was. I was raised in the
Midwest with a strong work ethic. I was taught that if you're not
bleeding, you're not actually hurt, and if you are bleeding, just rub
some dirt on it and it'll be fine. Anything that involved sitting still for
long periods ran contrary to my nature. If I wasn't actively doing
something, I was wasting my time. I had no interest in being lazy.

After my heart attack, I read a ton of articles and a lot of books
about health, particularly focused on the brain and mental health. I
was trying to find something, ANYTHING, that would help with my
anxiety, my headaches, and my lack of motivation. Meditation was
mentioned repeatedly as something that would help. I realized it was
time to overcome my bias against it, which required admitting I might
have been wrong about it.

Mindfulness falls into the same category as meditation, sort of like the little brother. Entire industries have been built around both. Each can be as complex as you make them.

I didn't realize it, but I'd been practicing mindfulness for years. As an IT consultant, I have been involved in several disaster recovery efforts. When computer systems go down because the servers crash, the organization is stopped in its tracks. Business stops. People stop getting paid. Everyone goes insane. The stress is unbelievable, but it was my job to recover the systems and bring the organization back online, as close to "normal" as possible.

Most of the time, I brought the systems back unscathed, but there were times I had to do a complete rebuild. In those cases, there was always a pivotal moment in which I had to decide to stop trying to fix the existing system and restore from the backup instead, to begin a total rebuild. The stress involved in making that decision is enormous. It wasn't just mental, but a physical weight I could feel pressing down on my body. I had to have faith that the customer's backup would work, because if it didn't, the data would be lost and the business would be crippled. In that moment, I felt genuine terror. A dialogue box will pop up to ask, "Do you wish to restore?" Answering "yes" begins the restore process, a point of no return.

I always paused before I pushed that button. I closed my eyes, I took a deep breath, and then I said the same prayer each time: "Dear Lord, please help me make the right decisions."

I would reflect on whether it was best to move forward with the restoration or continue my attempts at recovery.

That moment, in a nutshell, was mindfulness.

Mindfulness is a pause in which you pull yourself out of whatever situation you're in, reflect for a few moments, take a breath, gather yourself, and then take the next step. Mindfulness experts say it's important to adopt a nonjudgmental mentality.

It doesn't need to be complex. It doesn't require an app. Mindfulness is a simple tool you use to stop whatever is happening for a moment in time so you can reflect and be self-aware. That momentary pause can induce a sense of physical calm, giving you the courage to continue.

To me, meditation is just a longer, more complex form of mindful-ness. I'm sure there are many forms of meditation, but I don't need it to be complex. Meditation is an advanced form of mindfulness. I'll stick with that.

I wanted to learn about mindfulness and meditation because I was searching for anything that would help me calm my mind. I've had a restless mind most of my life. I've juggled multiple customers, projects, and a host of side gigs since I was a young man. I've been a writer my entire life. Sleep has never come easy for me because I just can't quiet my mind.

After my heart attack and brain injury, I quickly understood that if I was to make the fullest possible recovery, I would have to figure out how to give my mind the rest it needed.

I kept hearing about mindfulness, but I needed a place to start. I checked out books from the library, but they seemed to all start in the same unhelpful way:

"Find a peaceful place, a safe space, a quiet place. Withdraw your-self from everyone and everything around you."

If I had a safe, quiet, peaceful place with no one else around, why the hell would I need mindfulness? The same can be said for prayer. Anyone can pray when everything is quiet. I needed to learn how to be calm, to pray, to be mindful amid complete chaos. I needed a method to shut out the world and put my mind at rest while mayhem was going on around me.

I thought I knew what it meant to rest, but I didn't really under-stand that it meant turning off your mind, until I attended speech ther-apy. I always thought resting simply meant doing something that wasn't mentally taxing. My job can be mentally taxing, but I thought reading a novel could be considered "rest" because it didn't require much mental effort. My SLP explained that my mind was still active, processing the plot and characters of the book. Rest means doing noth-ing, putting the mind in a state of complete calm.

She taught me how to do this. She told me to close my eyes and focus on my breathing. I was to breathe in through my nose, then exhale slowly through my mouth. To calm the mind, I should aim for "belly breathing" instead of "chest breathing." Good belly breathing makes you fat while inhaling, then skinny while exhaling. I tried the technique a few times, and it was surprisingly calming. Next, I was to count my breaths as I inhaled and exhaled. She told me to practice at home. She challenged me to take a ten-minute break every hour.

My SLP had introduced me to mindfulness and a simple form of meditation. I didn't object to it as goofy or weird because I was desperate for anything that could help me get back to normal (or as close to normal as I could get). It also helped that she hadn't called it "mindfulness" or "meditation," which probably would have raised my bias shield. I would have been stubborn and unwilling to learn, and I'd have missed out on a technique that has been very effective in reclaiming my life.

I practiced the breathing technique at home. I tried to practice at work. The calming effect didn't work immediately; it took time and intentional effort before it began to help. I started by paying closer attention to my level of mental fatigue. When I felt it getting worse, I took a break and spent a few minutes doing the breathing technique.

Another popular breathing technique is called "box breathing" or "four-square breathing." Its beauty is in its simplicity. If you're a visual learner, there are many videos on the technique available on YouTube.

To begin, inhale through the nose. Count to four while you do this. By the time you reach four, your lungs should be full.

Hold your breath for a count of four. Count at the same pace at which you inhaled.

Exhale for a count of four.

Hold again for a count of four.

Repeat the process for five minutes.

It sounds simple, but it takes practice to get the timing down. You can do this with your eyes open or closed. It will be more calming and effective with your eyes closed, but if you are too anxious to close your eyes, it's okay to leave them open. You don't have to "assume a position," but it's best if you make yourself comfortable.

Over time, I discovered that I felt replenished if I rested periodically rather than trying to "power through" whatever I was working on, like I had done my entire life.

After a few months, I had learned to calm myself so well that I'd fall asleep while practicing the breathing techniques. I'd begin by counting my breaths, and I'd be asleep before I got to ten.

I'd take a ten- to fifteen-minute nap, wake up, and feel like a new person. It was very refreshing. My mental energy returned, my headaches lessened, and I could feel the stress melt away.

It's important to note that this process took a few months. This is an exercise that takes practice and patience to polish. Given that good sleep is the best thing I can do to ensure I have a good day, the practice was worthwhile.

For me, a nap should be no longer than twenty minutes. Ten minutes is ideal and easily achieved, but anything longer than twenty minutes does more harm than good. If I nap for an hour or two, I wake up feeling groggy and lethargic. Resting for that long is no longer a "nap," it's full-blown "sleep." Deep sleep is different from napping and should be saved for the end of the day.

I've concluded that the art of the ten-minute nap is a very advanced form of meditation.

How I Mastered the Ten-Minute Nap

To ready myself for a ten-minute nap,

I lay on my side on my bed or couch. I pull my legs up a little, but I don't go fully into the fetal position. I lay my head on a pillow and position both of my hands in a "prayer position" beneath my face. I focus on my breathing. I close my eyes. Then I inhale slowly through my nostrils and exhale slowly through my mouth. I count each breath.

When you give it a try, focus on your breath and counting. Also, remember to breathe with your abdomen, focusing on getting "fat and skinny." Typically, by the time I get to ten, I am asleep.

It didn't work for me right away. It took practice for me to improve my breathing technique and tune out distractions. I wish I'd looked into meditation or mindfulness years ago; I could've rid myself of all those sleepless nights with a racing mind.

This works well if you're somewhere where it's acceptable to fall asleep. But how can you calm your mind at work, where sleeping isn't an option?

You can use the same technique for calming your mind and giving yourself a reset. Simply sit in your chair with your body relaxed, your feet flat on the floor, close your eyes, and start focusing on your breathing. Again, breathe from your belly. Count your breaths and stop when you get to ten. Don't attempt to go to sleep, just focus on relaxing your body and quieting your mind. I've fallen asleep at customer sites, but my customers understand my recovery process and have been very accommodating.

The Beauty of Noise-Canceling Headphones

If you cannot make it through a full workday without becoming physically or mentally drained, prioritizing breaks at work is crucial to your recovery. You must be your own advocate. I am lucky to have excellent support from everyone around me. I am very vocal about what I need to do my job successfully; if I need everyone to be quiet or leave me alone, I explicitly ask. I am also willing to withdraw from work for a brief period to take a break.

You can't assume others will understand what you're going through if you don't tell them.

If I'm working on a tough problem, loud background sounds or people talking make it hard to concentrate and rapidly increase my mental fatigue. If I'm working in my home office, it isn't hard for me to shut out the world. I can turn off my cell phone, silence the notifications on my computer, and hide, if that's what it takes.

If I'm working at a customer site, it's much more difficult to find silence. To solve this problem, I carry noise-canceling headphones with me wherever I go. My entire work life is contained within a laptop bag. In addition to my computer, my bag includes over-ear headphones, Apple AirPods, and earplugs.

When I put on noise-canceling headphones, the world around me disappears. I listen to "focus" music on my phone. The best music for me is anything without singing or an upbeat tempo. There is an enormous selection of this type of music available on YouTube and Spotify. Search for "focus," and there are many playlists to choose from. I've discovered that I like beat-like electronic music best. It will take some experimentation to find one that's right for you.

Another option is to search for "binaural," which will lead you into the binaural beat world. Binaural beats play at specific frequencies to help you with focus, aid sleep, decrease anxiety, or increase relaxation, depending upon the frequency you choose. Personally, I have not experienced the magic others claim to have found in them, but they do block out background noise and distractions while I am working on complex problems.

Sometimes I listen to video game music. *Skyrim* and *Far Cry 4* both have soundtracks that I've enjoyed, and there are several others. Listening to that music transports me inside the game, another way of making the real world disappear momentarily. It doesn't matter how silly the music choice may seem to others as long as it works for you.

I have a pair of both Bose and Beats headphones.

They fit over the ear, so they are VERY noticeable. That's part of the point of wearing them. When customers see me wearing them, they know I am not to be disturbed as I am focusing on their problem. Not only do the headphones serve as a big signal, but I am also not shy about telling them. It is a natural impulse to want to hide our injuries, but when it comes to getting things done, I am very vocal about my needs. You must be your own advocate. If you aren't, you stand a greater chance of being run over by other people.

I use Apple AirPods when I want to be less obvious. They're still noticeable, since they're white, but they aren't as obnoxiously apparent as headphones. They can be used in noise-canceling or transparency mode. Noise-canceling mode shuts out the outside world, while transparency mode allows you to hear everything around you more easily.

When it's not feasible to use headphones or AirPods, I grab my earplugs. I try to avoid the cheap styrofoam earplugs and instead buy the ones used by musicians or people who ride motorcycles. My favorite brands are Eargasm and Vibes, but you should try several types to find the ones that work best for you. Earplugs can cut down on load noise while maintaining clarity, which can be enormously helpful at sporting events or places where many people are talking simultaneously. They are nonintrusive, so people don't notice me wearing them.

Specific Steps to Avoid Anxiety

When I feel myself getting anxious, I follow two very simple steps:

1. I close my eyes.
2. I focus on my breathing.

I work to shut out every external stimulus. I breathe in through my nose and out through my mouth. I pay attention to the air flowing in through my nostrils and into my chest. Sometimes I place my hand on my belly to feel it expand.

If I don't feel like I'm taking control, I do one of two things:

- I change my routine to breathe in and out of my mouth. I pay attention to how the air is cold when it enters my mouth and hot when it comes out.
- I continue to breathe in through my nose and out of my mouth, but I count my breaths, one count for each round trip in and out. I am calm by the time I reach ten.

Finally, I think about the good things in my life:

My beautiful wife, Heidi. Our kids. Our dog, Esther. I remember the last thing that made me laugh, the last good joke I heard, or maybe even the last good joke I told. I think about a place I'd like to visit or somewhere I've been that I would like to visit again. Imagining myself doing the activities I love, such as photography or fishing, can help me remove myself from the moment.

. . .

The point of these steps is to disrupt anxiety and quiet my mind. Anxiety can come on like a train barreling down the tracks, and you're tied to the rails. Your goal with mindfulness or meditation is to stop that train before it gets to you.

These steps likely won't work the first time you try them, or even the first five times. They are like exercise; they have to be done repeatedly before you hone the skill enough to see results.

Letting Negativity Go

Approaching mindfulness with a nonjudgmental mentality is incredibly important.

I've learned just how essential it is to manage your energy after a heart attack. Many trauma survivors experience mental fatigue, even those who don't have a traumatic brain injury. Everyday tasks take us longer and wear us out faster. I quickly realized that if I wanted to make the most of my life, I had to control my mental fatigue, which required an honest examination of the situations that sucked the most energy.

Through journaling, I discovered a huge number of day-to-day issues. After identifying the culprits, I sorted through them to determine whether they were things I could control, things that were important and unavoidable, or things I could just throw away.

This exercise helped me understand how much energy negative emotions consume. If I feel angry with someone, it drains my energy at an enormous rate. When I get frustrated at work, that frustration exhausts me. I realized I could preserve my much-needed mental energy if I threw those negative emotions away.

I began by calming myself, then dismissing the negative feelings. Later, I realized that I didn't have to work to dismiss them if I didn't acknowledge them in the first place. This had a feedback loop effect. I became a calmer person because I batted away anger at the onset, like having a force shield around me.

Life is tough. It's tougher after trauma. It's tougher still if I allow the world to drain my much-needed energy. I need that energy to recover, to lead the best life I can. I cannot afford to throw it away on negativity.

Anger is a barrier to recovery. My attitude toward recovery directly relates to how well and how quickly I can reclaim my life.

CHAPTER 11
JOURNALING

I ORIGINALLY STARTED JOURNALING BECAUSE I WANTED TO HAVE A BETTER understanding of my health. I wanted to track how often I had odd pains, and if they were dependent upon how well I slept, my diet, or how I felt overall. I finish my daily walk by going up a long, large hill, and I always noted what my heart rate was at the top of the hill. I tracked my heart rate when I biked through the spring and summer of 2020.

Keeping track of your health provides an ongoing account of where you've been and where you're going. It provides emotional release. I have found journaling to be an extremely useful tool in the fight against anxiety and depression. Thinking and writing about my day, including the things that bothered me, allows me to address them in a personal and nonjudgmental manner.

Journaling is the act of regularly writing your thoughts and feelings down to better understand them. It was once called "keeping a diary," but that conjures images of teenage girls in their bedroom, writing in a notebook protected by a cheesy lock. "Journaling" sounds much more mature than "keeping a diary," doesn't it? There is an entire industry built around journaling; Amazon offers a wealth of fancy books with writing prompts so you can journal in style.

I use a journal to write about all aspects of my life. I try to write every day. It has been immensely useful in determining what affects my health. I've tracked my sleep, diet, activities, and how I feel emotionally and physically. I used journaling to write my book, *Been Dead, Never Been To Europe*. Writing the book was cathartic; it helped me put my death behind me so I could move on and live life on my terms.

I journal about my goals. I keep track of what I did at work each day. This written record helps me remember why I made a decision or how we determined the parameters of an IT project. When customers ask questions about our project, I refer to my notes for a definitive answer.

I journal about what I'm grateful for. Gratitude journaling is a great way to turn bad thoughts to good. It helps to rewire your brain so you stop focusing on negative thoughts and start thinking about the good things in your life.

I journal about whatever is bothering me. Just the simple act of putting the words on paper helps me release the burden I'm feeling.

One good thing about journaling is that it's pretty close to free. Sure, you can invest in a leather-bound journal and fancy pens, but you can also buy a simple spiral notebook for your daily entries. You can write on your computer or use mobile apps designed for journaling. I prefer to do what I call, "voice journaling," where I talk into my cell phone. My voice is converted to text, and then I download the text into a journaling app.

I used journaling as a substitute for therapy. It helped me gain control of my anxiety and depression to such a degree that I didn't feel the need for personalized counseling. If your anxiety or depression is overwhelming, consider seeing a professional. I know people who wouldn't talk to a therapist if their life was in danger. I am still surprised at the number of people who don't understand that anxiety, depression, and stress can cause serious problems with their physical well-being.

Getting Started

You don't need a lot of equipment to get started with journaling; your preferred writing instrument and a simple notebook will do. Set aside ten to twenty minutes in your day to write in a notebook, and pledge to do it four or five days in a row.

Start by writing about a topic that is personal and important to you. Be sure to capture both the emotions and the event. The two are intertwined, and if you want to reap the most benefit, you're going to have to revisit the event.

Don't force it if you feel overwhelmed. In that case, it might be best to start on a less emotional subject and work your way to your trauma.

Write continuously for ten to twenty minutes without worrying about grammar, spelling, or structure. Don't worry about what your high school English teacher would think. Don't worry about what your family, your friends, or your pastor would think. This journal is for you. It is not for anyone else to read unless you allow it. You can even destroy what you've written after you're finished, but it can be beneficial to reread your entry later to remind yourself of where you were at the time of writing.

Accept that starting is going to be difficult. You're likely to experience a rush of emotion. It took me three years to write *Been Dead, Never Been To Europe* because I cried every time I wrote or edited. By the end, I understood a lot more about who I am and where I'm going than I would have if I'd never written it. I still cry whenever I do an interview or talk about my trauma when meeting new people, and that's okay.

Expect to feel sad. Trauma is damn hard. Dealing with the emotional fallout of trauma is hard. "Hard" should not be a reason to avoid growth. Burying and ignoring those emotions will only ensure that they will linger, then fester, then boil over, probably at the worst possible time. Emotions rarely explode when you're alone at home. Instead, they explode when all the other stress in your life spins out of control. When the dam finally bursts, the people you love most are typically standing directly in the path of the water. You're left wondering how to clean up the mess you've made.

Don't do that. Try journaling instead. You can do it alone in your bathroom if you like. Stick a towel in your mouth if you're worried about others hearing you cry. (Gee, it's almost as if I've been there.) You have my permission.

You may find it difficult to get started with the actual writing if you're not ready to jump right into your traumatic event. What should you write about? What should you say?

You can start by asking yourself the following questions:

- What's important to you?
- What are your goals?
- What worries you?
- What do you fear?
- What causes you anxiety?
- What do you want to do with your life?
- What are you thankful for?
- How do you spend most of your time?

If you're having problems getting started, imagine you're talking to an imaginary friend. They're not just for children. I pretend I'm talking to an alien, explaining life on this planet, human beings, and how screwy we are. Sometimes I pretend I'm talking to a real-life friend or loved one; I imagine them sitting next to me. I imagine I'm talking to my mom, who died in 2012. She always has the answers to my biggest questions. Mom is still a fountain of wisdom.

You can do the same. You can tell those people (or aliens) all the things you want to tell them, if you only could. Tell them in your private journal. You might find it easier to talk to them the next time you're presented with the opportunity.

Leading by Example

I believe in leading by example, so I'm going to provide my answer to one of the sample questions to help you get started. (In reality, I believe in leading by screaming profanities at people at the top of my lungs, but that won't work here.)

What's *important to me?*

Defining what's important allows me to set priorities. It's easy to get sidetracked, to spend hours on the internet going down the rabbit hole only to discover I've accomplished nothing all day. Arguing with strangers on the internet can be interesting and sometimes fun, but it's not important. It does nothing positive for me. Arguing doesn't help me meet my goals. In fact, it gets in the way. Most of the time, it just makes me angry, which takes my energy away.

Unfortunately, it's easy to get sucked into, which is why I define what's important, so I have a reference for what I wish to focus on.

The most important things in my life are:

My faith in God, which I will freely admit is not as strong as it should be. I am a Christian most of the time.

My family. I have an obligation to my wife to provide for her. I know myself well enough to know that if I can't be a provider, I will feel worthless. I have an obligation to my wife and kids to be a decent husband and father. I quit drinking because I was failing miserably at this part of my life. My wife and children deserve to have a husband and father who isn't a mess.

My customers. I am paid a decent wage to solve my customers' problems, to be dependable, and to provide value. I take that charge seriously.

My friends. They deserve to be treated with respect. They don't need me to overburden them with my issues, as they have their own. They need me to listen and be a decent human being.

My website and my writers. I run a sports website, and I have a full staff of writers who write for me. It's important that I treat them with dignity and respect, and provide them with opportunities to grow as writers while having fun doing it. It's important that I put them in a position to be successful.

Everything and everyone on this list take priority over everything else.

What I've Learned from Journaling

I have learned an immense amount about myself from journaling. Looking back, I realize that defining my goals and determining what's most important to me has helped me tremendously in my daily life. It helps me align myself with my goals, understand how to prioritize my time, and identify the best ways to protect my mental energy.

I spend an inordinate amount of time on the internet accomplishing nothing. Remembering my goals, I understand that time spent that way is wasted. I frequently ask myself if what I'm doing is important, if it's helping me get anywhere. If it isn't, I have to decide whether I want to continue wasting my time or stop what I'm doing. I know this sounds like I'm conducting a business seminar on productivity, and perhaps I am.

Focusing on what's important helps with my memory. Perhaps it's no surprise at this point, but I have strong opinions. They are reflected in my career, my writing, my podcasts, and my YouTube videos. I frequently receive very negative comments from people who disagree with me, particularly when I'm writing or talking about sports. They can be very insulting. I have learned to ignore them, which isn't that hard to do.

Are complete strangers who send nasty emails on the list of people I care about? No. Then why should I care about what they have to say about me? I let it go. I forget about it. (Well, I do my best to forget about it.)

Every once in a while, a negative comment will get to me. They stick me like a dagger, especially when they're right. Perhaps I said something stupid, and a commenter points out how stupid it was. I immediately think, "How could I have been so stupid?"

I get angry about it. The anger exhausts me. I can feel the energy drain from me, as if someone were draining the blood from my body. If I don't stop to reflect upon what's important, my headache pain will explode, and a single, meaningless comment will ruin my day.

The same philosophy applies to encounters in the real world. Perhaps the cashier at Target makes a comment I don't like. I get cut off in traffic. I want to relax on my deck, but my neighbor is having a loud party. The dog barks at everyone who walks by our house, sometimes even barking at nothing at all. I break my fancy French press coffee maker.

Although these situations are frustrating, they're not important in the end. They don't impede my goals. They're certainly not worth ruining my day over, so I do my best to forget them immediately. My ability to drop whatever angers me didn't happen overnight. I worked at it. It was like exercising; I had to train myself to let go.

If something happens that involves "The Important Group" and I can't resolve it, I journal about it. I ask myself why it bothers me, what I can do to fix it, and how I can do better in the future.

Another major benefit of journaling is that it helps me identify which habits affect my health. Tracking my health is how I learned that a good night of sleep is the single most beneficial thing I can do to ensure the least amount of chronic headache pain in the morning. I experiment on myself a lot. I've worked on tracking different supplements, such as magnesium, to determine how they affect my health.

Journaling has helped me better understand this process. Without it, I wouldn't be nearly as productive as I am.

It's as close to free therapy as I am going to get. The only actual cost is confronting myself and being open about who I am, where I'm going, and what I want for my life.

It's easy to get started, and it only takes twenty minutes a day. Journaling is truly one of the most beneficial strategies I've found in my recovery.

CHAPTER 12
SLEEP STRATEGIES

GETTING RESTFUL SLEEP IS ONE OF THE BEST THINGS I CAN DO FOR MY recovery. It's the biggest factor in whether I have a good day. Since sleep has never come easily for me, finding things that worked took a lot of trial and error.

Reliance on Alcohol

For years, I took the all-too-common path of drinking alcohol before bedtime, thinking it would help me fall asleep. In reality, all I accomplished was waking up with a hangover and feeling lethargic and damn near useless. I treated alcohol like a friend because I understood its behavior. I knew what to expect. If I drank myself to sleep, I wouldn't feel any better in the morning, but I told myself it was better than not sleeping at all. I had closed my mind to other options.

When I sobered up, the headache pain was overwhelming, so I'd start drinking again to relieve the pain. It was a footrace to hell. Even at the time, I could see how detrimental it was to my health, but I didn't see a way out of the vicious cycle.

Finally, in April 2020, I ended my alcohol consumption for good, and I have no intention of having it again.

. . .

Sleep Aids

In my desperation for sleep, I have tried sleeping pills. I awake groggy, and I remain groggy and lethargic for the rest of the day after I've taken them. The side effects are more detrimental than the pills are worth. They're like alcohol in that way. If you're interested in trying them, consult your doctor to verify they won't interact badly with the medication you're already taking.

Occasionally, I use melatonin when I want to fall asleep quickly. I've used melatonin supplements that include L-theanine, chamomile, zinc, magnesium, L-arginine and L-lysine. I've tried chamomile herbal tea, and an assortment of other teas.

None of these help me fall asleep any better than the routine I've developed.

A combination of melatonin with L-theanine seems to be helping me stay asleep longer. Lately, I have been using a supplement from Olly, "Sleep," which are gummies that contain melatonin, L-theanine, chamomile, passionflower, and lemon balm.

Sleeping Alone

I sleep in my own room. My wife and I have found that it's best for both of us and we get a better night's sleep than we would sleeping together.

We work different hours. Sleeping in my own room means that I don't wake her up when I come to bed later than her, and she doesn't wake me up when she gets up for work at four o'clock each morning.

I do miss the feeling of her warm body next to mine at night, especially in the winter. It's nice to wake up next to someone you love. Well, it would be nice if you get up at the same time. If they're waking you up early and you just went to bed, it really sucks.

The other big problem we had when we slept together were my dreams. I often have terrible dreams, and in the past, I have woken Heidi up with my screams or by punching or kicking her. Even without the punching and kicking, I frequently thrashed around the bed all night. The bed covers would be a mess and she would wake up exhausted. As much as I miss sharing a bed with my wife, we both get better sleep alone.

Weighted Blanket

I performed a home sleep study after a discussion with my family doctor to determine whether I had sleep apnea. It turned out that I don't, but he noted that I am very active in my sleep. I was relieved to learn that I don't have sleep apnea because I don't want to wear a Darth Vader mask every night.

I mentioned the doctor's comment about how I am "very active when sleeping" to Heidi. She suggested I try a weighted blanket. I had never heard of such a thing and wondered why anyone would voluntarily use a blanket that would hold them down. After she described the benefits, it sounded like a really good idea, so she picked one up for me.

It worked very well. I had no problem adjusting to its weight, and it really does help my body stay still at night, which leads to higher quality sleep. I don't use it in the summer because it makes me too hot, but it's especially great in the winter.

Sound

I have trained my brain using sound. I use sound to put myself to sleep every night, just like I've tried to create habits around exercise. Some sounds are naturally relaxing; waves crashing on the beach, heavy rain, and thunderstorms do it for me. The sound of the wind blowing through the trees reminds me of camping in a tent in the forest.

Using sound to train your brain for sleep is like most other strategies: it requires repetition. It didn't help me at first, but after a while, my brain got conditioned to associate the sound with feeling sleepy. It works so well that I could fall asleep writing this if I were to play those sounds. If I'm not careful, I'll be drooling on my keyboard.

· · ·

Avoiding Technology before Bed

The effect of blue light on our ability to sleep has gotten a lot of press lately. The sun emits blue light, as do fluorescent and incandescent light bulbs and devices that use LEDs, such as laptops, televisions, cell phones, and tablets.

Research shows that exposure to blue light suppresses the body's natural melatonin, disrupting a person's circadian rhythm, which is the body's internal clock that regulates the sleep-awake cycle.

I am still skeptical about the effects of blue light and the entire circadian rhythm concept. But since I'm very protective of my sleep, I use dark mode on my computer screens.

I also try to avoid electronics for thirty minutes before I go to bed, with the brief exception of starting the sleep app on my phone. So although I am skeptical, I have had really good results with this process.

Establish a Specific Process

I have experimented heavily in my search for perfect sleep. One key to falling asleep quickly is having a calm mind. Calming my mind through mindfulness and journaling has really benefited the overall quality of my sleep. It's important to establish a predictable routine. This consistency helps train your body to be ready for sleep.

I go to bed at the same time every night: midnight. I've tried going to bed earlier, but I'm never able to fall asleep before midnight. My goal is to wake up at six o'clock. I'd love to be able to sleep in for an extra couple of hours, but no matter how hard I've tried, I just cannot get a full eight hours of sleep.

Sometimes, I take melatonin before I go to bed, although I can go to sleep without it. It doesn't help with longevity of sleep. It can help you fall asleep, but it will not keep you asleep.

I lie on my back. I say my prayers, although I'm not as consistent with that as I'd like to be. I thank God for my wife, my children, and another day of life, in that order.

My mind should be calm.

In the past, this is the exact moment at which I would start thinking about the next day's work, ideas to write about, or some genius invention. My mind would be anything but calm, exploding with activity. If my mind isn't calm when I lie down, I either practice my breathing technique or read a book for a while to let my brain do some work. The key here is to control what my brain is doing rather than letting it run wild, ruminating on regrets or stressing over work.

When my mind has calmed, I move to the last step.

I launch the app on my phone that plays the sound of thunderstorms. When my brain hears that sound, it knows it's time to go to sleep. It doesn't matter if I'm ready to sleep for the night or I'm just taking a quick nap.

I use a body pillow to put myself in a comfortable position. I sleep on my side, so I turn over and throw one leg over the pillow. With a quiet mind, the sounds of a thunderstorm, a dark room, and a comfortable pillow, I am normally asleep within a couple of minutes.

Establishing a process is so important to falling asleep quickly. My mind and body know what to expect. This involves habit and training, which takes time. It doesn't work right away, but now I very rarely have trouble falling asleep.

CHAPTER 13
MEMORY

In this chapter, I'm going to talk about two types of memory: long-term and short-term memory. I do not intend to offer scientific definitions; rather, I'll discuss how my heart attack has impacted the two types of memory, and some strategies I've found to help.

My idea of short-term memory is whatever you need to remember to get through your day successfully, such as where you put your car keys, what you're going to work on, or what you hope to accomplish.

Long-term memory, on the other hand, involves anything you're expected to remember over weeks, years, or decades. This includes life skills, important events, important people in your life, and every piece of terrible dialogue from every *Star Wars* movie.

Short-Term Memory Strategies

When I first came home from the hospital, my short-term memory was nonexistent. It got better over time, but I still had to manage to get through life in the early weeks of my recovery. The strategies I use most often to cope with my lack of short-term memory are relying on technology and adopting a strict routine.

I carry a cell phone and wallet wherever I go. Since my cell phone is always with me, it's easy to create reminders, timers, and alarms about everything imaginable. I created recurring reminders to take my medication every morning and evening. Heidi later told me that she had to remind me to take my medicine for about a year after my heart attack. She managed my medication in one of those seven-day pill organizers, so if the pills were gone, she knew I took them. If a dose was left in the container, she knew I hadn't taken them, despite the reminder on my phone. Having someone to support and help me was indispensable in the first few months of my recovery.

I'm not shy about using technology. If I am grilling hamburgers, I will create a timer to check the grill in five minutes. I'll set an alarm on my Apple watch to check on the mac and cheese in eight minutes. If I'm doing laundry, I'll create a reminder to move my clothes from the washer to the dryer, then another reminder in a couple of hours to retrieve them from the dryer.

To set a reminder on my watch, I push the side button, then say, "Set a reminder to check the hamburgers in five minutes." It doesn't get much easier than that!

I embrace technology. That's what it's here for. When I was a kid, I remember the Dick Tracy cartoons in the newspaper; they were always talking to their watches on the two-way wrist TV. I thought it was the coolest thing ever. I'll be first in line to buy one when they invent the Air Car so I can fly around and talk to other people on my watch.

I use technology to organize and plan my life. There are myriad apps available for productivity and tracking to-do lists. I use these for the gobs of different activities I'm involved in. I often have several projects running concurrently at work. I need to track their progress and stay organized, or I'll get lost and spend time and effort trying to figure out where I was, which is both embarrassing and unproductive. I use these tools to supplement both my short- and long-term memory for projects that are single-day efforts or that last over a period of several months.

I have used technology to keep myself organized for two decades, long before my heart attack. I don't like using paper, since it can be easily lost or destroyed. Many people rely on handwritten journals and daily planners to get through their lives. I tried those things for a while, but my handwriting is terrible and it exacerbates the carpal tunnel and repetitive stress issues with my hands and wrists. I use technology whenever possible to keep track of everything in my life.

I use my cell phone to take photos of where I've parked. If I go to a sporting event, for example, I try to park in the same location every time. Even then, when I get out of my car, I take a photo of the nearest landmark. It might be the street signs at a corner or the sign on a parking ramp that shows what section I'm in. If I can't remember where I parked when the event is over, I can easily look at my phone and save myself the time spent wandering around aimlessly. I don't delude myself into thinking that I'll remember where I parked, because I know I won't. Besides, I don't want to rely on my memory when I have a device that can do that for me. It's not a weakness; it's an efficient use of my resources! I apply my superior use of technology for its purpose, then feel like I'm smarter than everyone else for doing it. That way I don't feel quite as bad about my crappy memory.

Heidi keeps a handwritten calendar on the door in our kitchen. I'm thankful it's there because it tells me what everybody else is doing throughout the month. I can easily check the family calendar against the calendar in my phone to avoid scheduling conflicts.

There are three things I need to keep track of at all times: my cell phone, wallet, and car keys. I'm diligent about returning each of these items to their assigned place.

We have a key rack on the wall right next to the door to our garage. The car keys are kept there for anybody who wants to use them. I don't carry a personal set of car keys. I pull the keys off the rack. They're attached to a lanyard that goes around my neck. I pull the keys and immediately put them around my neck. Then I get in the car, take the keys off, and start the car. After I've arrived and shut off the engine, the keys go back around my neck. When I come home, the first thing I do is put the keys back on the key rack. It's a consistent habit, practiced by everyone in our household. I never have to search for keys. I always know exactly where they are.

The same routine applies to my wallet. My wallet stays in one of three places: on a specific spot on my desk, in a specific pocket of my laptop bag, or in the breast pocket of my winter coat during the cold months. I never come home and toss my wallet somewhere random . . . Okay, sometimes I do. I'm not perfect, but those are the times it gets lost, and I get upset because I didn't follow my routine.

My cell phone goes wherever I go. It's always with me. It's not just my connection to the world, but it's also my connection to how I make a living. I need to be available whenever one of my customers has an emergency. If I lose my cell phone, it's the end of the world, or at least the end of my income, which might be the same thing.

Long-Term Memories

I have spent an exceptional amount of energy lamenting my lost memories. Finally, I had to face the truth that I'll never get them back. There was no magic, no revisiting places or reliving events that would make a difference. They were gone.

I felt terrible about it, but then I realized I'd be better off if I stopped trying to recover the past and focused instead on the future. I want to make new memories instead of crying about the old ones. I decided to move on. Just like making a decision to be happy, I made the choice to let the past go. I didn't forget everything on purpose, nor do I avoid hearing about my past when it comes up, but I no longer attempt to recover lost memories or ruminate about them. Feeling sorry for myself about the loss of a lifetime of memories only makes me melancholy. I don't want to live that way anymore. Enough is enough.

The same is true for life skills I've forgotten. As a Boy Scout leader, I learned and taught knot tying, orienteering, CPR, and outdoor survival skills. I've forgotten so much of what I used to know. Now, I couldn't tie a bowline knot if I were forced. A clove hitch or a taut line are out, and tying a double sheet bend is just as difficult as discovering how to use wormholes to navigate the universe.

I could relearn them, but they are no longer relevant to my everyday life. No one wants me to go out into the wilderness for fun anymore. I might die on them and they'd have to haul my body back, which would be a miserable experience because they wouldn't know the knots necessary to build a makeshift stretcher.

When I died, I lost a lot of the memories I had of books and movies. I have been a voracious reader all my life. Over the years, I collected a lot of quotes from books as a way of supplementing my memory. If I read the quote, I can remember what key points I took away from the book. Now, most of the time, I look at those quotes and have no recollection of having ever read that book. I lost the memories of most of the sci-fi books I've read over the years. I've chosen to reread a few, but I'm not as captivated by future visions of science as I was when I was young. However, I am seasoned enough to appreciate not just the story but the writing as a craft. Rereading an old story is a different, beautiful, brand new experience.

Over the years, my family has made a habit of acting out scenes from movies. We'd be eating dinner when someone would say a line, then everyone else would follow up with the rest of the scene. Since most of my movie memories have evaporated, I'm lost most of the time now. It's frustrating because it's fun and I feel left out.

I didn't lose my memory of music. I can hear a song from my youth that I haven't heard in twenty years and still remember it, the lyrics, everything.

Making New Long-Term Memories

There are many books, websites, and courses on how to build a super impressive long-term memory. They all use similar techniques. There's the "Memory Palace" technique, where you associate what you want to remember with a location you're familiar with, like your house. This is particularly useful when you want to memorize a list of items. As you visualize yourself walking through your house, you associate the objects you want to remember with objects that exist in your house. The more colorful you make the association, the better your retention. When the time comes to remember the list, you take a mental tour of your palace to recall the associations.

The memory palace technique requires a huge amount of mental processing. I couldn't use it again if I tried. I would be too fatigued to even set it up in my mind.

Another technique is to create an acronym of what you want to remember, or to make up a rhyme. For example, one thing I remember about the bowline knot is the rhyme we used to teach it: "Up through the rabbit hole, round the big tree; down through the rabbit hole and off goes he." We would recite that rhyme while demonstrating how to tie the knot. Despite my widespread memory loss, I still remember the rhyme. I don't remember the knot, but maybe I could tie the knot by following the rhyme.

I read books and watched YouTube videos on improving my memory. Rather than helpful solutions, I was treated to people telling me I wasn't listening hard enough. I was told there's no such thing as having a good memory or bad memory, only trained memories and untrained memories. I was told I would be terrible at business if I didn't remember the names of everyone I'd ever met. I'd be publicly shunned.

The people who come up with these solutions pride themselves on being able to remember the names of thirteen billion people, despite the fact that there's only a little less than eight billion people on earth.

Each one of the memory techniques I examined had one commonality: they all required mental effort. In order to remember someone's name, I was supposed to associate them with an object. I had to make a mental effort to create that association. When I see them again, I'm supposed to recall the association and therefore the name.

All this mental effort requires energy. Specifically, it requires brain energy. Fatigue remains one of the most frustrating aspects of my life. I get tired when I work physically, but I get even more fatigued from mental processing. Just trying to implement any of these memory techniques wore me out.

I was disappointed by how poor my memory was until it occurred to me to ask, "Why do I need to remember all this stuff in the first place?"

I realized that I was wasting so much energy remembering things that weren't important. Now, I focus on the people and things on my Important List, and those are the only things I commit to long-term memory. Those are the only things I worry about day to day. I don't care about remembering the capital of Vermont or what year the Magna Carta was signed. They are unimportant. I don't care which German U-boat sank the *Lusitania*. I can look it up. I would fail miserably in a trivia competition, so I just don't apply to be on game shows. Problem solved.

If I go to a nice restaurant and have a delicious meal, I don't bother remembering what I ate. If I think it might be memorable, I take a photo before I eat. Is remembering what I ate at a nice restaurant important? No. I enjoy the meal in the moment and then I move on with my life. Eating an enjoyable meal isn't among the things I defined as important, so I don't commit it to memory.

I don't use part of my brain's processing power to commit things to memory that aren't important to me. It may seem like a small effort to remember those things, but each one contributes to the fatigue I deal with every day, everywhere, all the time. Combating fatigue is more important than remembering the trivial things I encounter in life.

I purposefully don't work to remember all the things I did throughout the day. I don't remember letting our dog Esther out or taking her for a walk. I don't care. Esther will let me know if she needs to go out. It will be okay.

What about bigger life events that are more important, such as my children's birthdays? Those are trickier. My youngest son, Isaiah, recently had a birthday and asked me how old I thought he was. I guessed. I was wrong. I could tell by the look on his face that he was disappointed in me. I was off by a year, but remembering what day they were born or how old my kids are isn't as important to me as remembering what they're doing with their lives. He just graduated from the University of Minnesota with a math degree. That's more important to me than knowing how old he is. (If this sounds like a sorry dad excuse, you're right. It is.)

This can sometimes be embarrassing. I was recently at a sporting event and a person I'd met two years before came up to say hello. We work together over email every once in a while, but I didn't remember his face. I'd forgotten what he looked like. It was a little embarrassing, but again, not that important. It sounds rude, but this is the price I pay for recovery.

The reality of my life after my heart attack is that I have to choose between avoiding mental fatigue or remembering everybody I encounter in my life. To maximize the quality of my life, I choose to avoid fatigue.

I rely on technology quite heavily to support my long-term memory. I frequently use my phone's camera to take photos of places I've been. If I see the photo, I can more easily remember what happened on that occasion. This isn't hugely different from my life before my heart attack. I've carried a camera around for most of my life, and I've taken thousands of photos over the years. I enjoy photography, but now I also use it as a memory strategy.

Events I want to remember go into my digital calendar, accessible and shared between my laptop, my desktop computer, and the cell phone that's always with me. My journal records my life. If I want to recall a day or an event that happened, I can search my journal.

If it sounds like I'd be lost without technology, it's only partially true. I am involved in quite a huge number of activities because I can lean on technology to track everything. If I lost those tools, my life would shrink.

CHAPTER 14
MEDICATION

In the early days of my recovery, I did what I was told and took the medication I was given without question. I tried to learn what each of the pills did for me, but my mental capacity was terrible. My cardiologist explained my regimen repeatedly, but it was utterly confusing. I couldn't understand that there were several names for each drug. The label on my pill bottle would read clopidogrel, but then I'd go to the pharmacist and they'd mention Plavix. They could have given me whatever they wanted, and I'd have taken it because I thought that was the best way to recover.

Over the years, I have become much more vigilant about understanding what I'm taking. I have a strong desire not to take anything, so if I'm prescribed a drug, there had better be an excellent reason for it. I don't distrust my doctors, particularly my cardiologist. He has been an excellent doctor. I feel comfortable having very blunt discussions with him, particularly about the medication he's prescribing. Everything I take has a pretty clear goal: helping me avoid another heart attack. They aren't magical, they aren't guaranteed to keep it from happening. They simply reduce the risk. We discuss the risks and whether the benefits justify taking the medication. In the end, I ask him for his recommendation and typically follow it because I trust his judgment.

When I started taking my medication, I wish I had asked the doctor what to do about missing a dose. I'd never experienced something as traumatic and life altering as my heart attack, so I was unaccustomed to having to take medication regularly. In the beginning, I wondered if missing a dose would kill me. Then I wondered if taking two doses to make up for the missed dose would kill me. It turned out not to be a big deal, but I should have asked my doctors about it when they first prescribed the medicine.

In my never-ending quest to deal with fatigue, I have blamed several of my medications for it. After discussions with my cardiologist, I have experimented with the types of medication and the dosages to see if I can identify the cause of my fatigue. So far, I am averaging zero.

Statins have a terrible reputation for causing a variety of side effects. I have taken atorvastatin (Lipitor) for years. After I complained one too many times, my cardiologist finally agreed to let me discontinue it to see if it caused my fatigue. It was not the culprit. The same was true for metoprolol and clopidogrel, both medicines I took earlier in my recovery.

The reason I know the statins aren't responsible for my fatigue is because of my diligent journaling. When I change a drug, my diet, my sleep habits, or my exercise routine, I keep track of how I feel in my journal.

The most prominent side effect I experienced with the statins wasn't fatigue, but muscle cramps. I've never had cramps in my feet, let alone in the middle of the night, before taking a statin. I never realized how painful foot cramps can be. The cramps were significantly reduced when I added CoQ10 to my regimen.

I am hesitant to look up the side effects for my medication because I know it will influence how I feel about taking it. Medical Student Syndrome occurs when people who are working to become doctors begin to believe they are experiencing the symptoms of the disease they're studying. Up to 70 percent of medical students are affected by this malady.

If medical students can be so easily influenced by what they're reading, what chance do I stand when I go onto internet forums to read about the terrible experiences of others?

I have been blessed to have a knowledgeable, compassionate team of doctors assisting me in my recovery. I have always felt that they have my best interest at heart. I know I can sometimes be a handful, but not a single one of them has ever acted as if they didn't want to talk to me, care for me, or give me the best advice possible.

Be your own advocate and find doctors you trust. Be sure they explain why they recommended the medication you're taking. If you have questions about side effects, ask. Ask for guidance about what to do if you miss a dose. Be sure you understand which symptoms can be waited out at home, and which symptoms warrant a trip to the hospital. If you're experiencing pain or other trouble, be honest and transparent. If you find your doctor to be off-putting or unwilling to explain, find a different doctor.

CHAPTER 15
POSITIVE THINKING

I SPENT MY SHARE OF TIME FEELING SORRY FOR MYSELF. AFTER MY HEART attack, I lamented all the things I'd no longer be able to do. For most of my life, I always enjoyed spending my vacation time in the middle of nowhere, camping, hunting, and fishing. After my heart attack, I was sure I'd never get to do those things again. I love photography, but because of my brain injury, I wasn't sure I'd remember how to properly use a camera.

Then there was the problem of memory. Huge chunks of my life had just vanished from my mind. Listening to my family talk about vacations we'd taken together but not remembering anything about them hurt tremendously. I wasn't as concerned about my own childhood memories, but losing the memories of when my children were little was incredibly painful.

I got stuck in the "Why me?" period of recovery. I wallowed.

It's okay to allow ourselves periods of self-pity. What's not okay is allowing it to take over your life or prevent you from being the person you want to be or doing what you want to do. There's no point in dwelling on the pre-trauma life you had.

I had to convince myself that I still have a lot of life yet to experience. I have no desire to feel sorry for myself for the rest of my life. The life I had before my heart attack is gone. I have tried to tell myself it is okay to create new memories to replace those that are gone.

Yet, there I was, stuck on that question of "Why?"

The best way I've found to get out of that rut is to turn your bad thoughts into good. It's not easy, but it's a game changer. Rather than sitting around, thinking about your trauma, think about what you want to do with your life instead.

Turning bad thoughts to good works in conjunction with mindfulness. If you feel yourself ruminating on a negative thought, especially one you can't change, you can use mindfulness to pull yourself back, still your thoughts, and then think of something positive to replace the bad thoughts you're having.

Whenever I slip back into "why me" mode, I think about the good in my life. I have a beautiful wife who loves me after thirty years of marriage. I have three adult children and I am still around to watch them grow. I enjoy writing. I enjoy podcasting, ranting like a lunatic about sports on YouTube, and doing photography. I have never written a novel, but I'd like to write one someday.

When I'm stuck in a rut, I try to come up with stories I'd like to write, people I'd like to interview on a podcast, or stupid YouTube videos I want to make. I fancy myself a content creator, so I am constantly trying to think up ideas for articles, photos, and videos.

To help me take stock of the good in life, I go outside and look at the world around me. I marvel at how beautiful it is: the way the light comes through the trees, the clouds, the life flourishing all around. Our world is incredibly beautiful if you take a moment to notice.

Gratitude journaling is an excellent way to establish the habit of thinking good thoughts. The idea is to identify five or ten things you're grateful for every day. It's easy to say that you're grateful for your spouse or kids, but challenge yourself! Change it up every day, even if you're especially appreciative of the really great cup of coffee you had one morning.

One of the best ways to forget about my own troubles is doing something I enjoy. When I am immersed in an activity, I can ignore my headaches and troubles. If I'm not doing something that brings me joy, I am much more aware of how badly my back aches or how badly my head is throbbing. The key is finding a way to keep my brain active and focused on something other than myself.

If I go to an event, such as a football game, a play, or a movie, I become so engrossed by what's going on that I completely forget about myself for a while.

Another way of focusing on the positive is to do charity work or volunteer for an organization. I spent years involved with coaching kids' soccer and being a Boy Scout leader. If I lived one thousand more lives, I would volunteer to do that again one thousand more times. There's nothing like helping others to make you grateful for the good things in your life.

Try to avoid stress or anxiety-producing situations. This might be as simple as staying away from social media. We all have certain sites or topics that can make us angry, and anger is exhausting. Try avoiding those sites for a while. Keep a journal and see how different you feel over time. You obviously can't avoid everything difficult or stressful, but making a concerted effort to cut down on stress will help you break free from negativity until it becomes a habit.

Like meditation, turning your bad thoughts to good won't work the first ten times you do it. It takes practice. You must train yourself to recognize when you're falling into the well of misery, then take steps— like stepping outside to look at the trees, the light, the clouds—to pull yourself out of that darkness.

It took me months to establish positive thinking as a habit. Now, I very rarely ask myself "Why?" I am in control of my anxiety and depression. Moments of anxiety still happen, but they don't last very long. I can push them away much more quickly than I could before because I know the good things in my life outweigh the bad.

CHAPTER 16
FINDING PURPOSE

AT SOME POINT IN THEIR LIVES, EVERYONE HAS ASKED THEMSELVES, "WHY am I here?" Great minds have established entire branches of philosophy in an attempt to answer that question. College kids ponder their existence as they stare into the next forty years of loyal servitude to whatever corporate entity they decide to serve. Those determined to be self-employed wake up in the middle of the night wondering if they'll make payroll, while simultaneously asking, "Why am I doing this?" A spouse may wonder why they are left to assume the roles they thought their partner would take on.

"Why" is a universal question that haunts us, no matter our race, religion, identity, or location on the planet.

When we're young, we're determined to change the world. As we get older, we grow cynical and we realize there is no changing the world. You might move it a few degrees, but when most of us hit fifty, we just want to get out of bed in the morning without feeling like hell.

Questioning your existence becomes much greater when you experience trauma. Maybe you're in a car accident. You're run over while biking. You overdose but survive. You're diagnosed with cancer. Confronted with your own mortality, you reflect on your life and conclude that there must be some great deed you must accomplish to make it all worthwhile.

Not long after I came home from the hospital, two other men from my community suffered severe heart attacks and died. Both were under fifty years old. Both left young children behind.

In 2017, I lost a great friend, Brian, to complications with his heart. He had gone into the hospital with blood clots in his lungs. He was so adamant about getting back to work. I kept trying to tell him to relax and that everything was okay. I told him that he should take care of himself. That was the last thing I ever said to him.

I woke up the next morning to five missed phone calls from his wife. I knew what had happened. When I returned her call, she shared the sad news that a blood clot had broken loose and moved into his heart. The hospital staff performed CPR on him for an hour, but they couldn't bring him back. He was only forty-one years old. He left behind a sixteen-year-old son and a three-year-old daughter. I went to his funeral and watched his daughter try to wake him up to give him a stuffed toy. She kept screaming at her daddy to wake up and get out of the coffin. It was the most difficult experience I've ever had in my life.

Why am I still here when those children lost their fathers?

The experience drove me to believe that I must accomplish a monumental task to justify my life. There had to be a reason I had survived. I looked for it everywhere. I secretly hoped disaster would strike so I could prove myself to be a hero. Maybe I could save someone from a car accident, pull a family from a burning house, or put myself in danger so others could escape an active shooter. My TED Talk, which I'm sure will come any day, would make the world a better place.

This devotion to finding a great accomplishment kept me awake at night. It became madness. I stopped living my regular life for a while, certain I could find a way to make up for surviving something that should have killed me. After a while, I realized I had to let it go and fall back to the one grand purpose for which we are all created.

In the 2001 movie *Moulin Rouge*, Toulouse-Lautrec, played beautifully by John Leguizamo, declares,

. . .

"The greatest thing you'll ever learn is just to love and be loved in return."

This pronouncement comes just as the movie reaches its fateful, tragic, love-filled climax.

It perfectly encompasses the purpose that guides my life: love. (The line originated from the Nat King Cole song, "Nature Boy," but writers can't quote lyrics anywhere without being attacked by lawyers, so screw you, music industry.)

It's been six years since I died. In the time since, I've taught myself to let everything unimportant or negative go. I don't hold grudges because I don't remember the people or the event about which I should be angry. As it turns out, it's pretty easy to forgive and forget if you practice it daily.

Letting go allows me to focus on what matters: my faith, my wife, my kids, my friends, my job, and my health.

I do my best to let those around me know that I love them, and I know they love me in return.

That is enough for a healthy, fulfilled life.

CHAPTER 17
DEALING WITH TRAUMA ANNIVERSARIES

I died on August 21, 2015. What else happened on August 21 throughout history? I don't know. I had to look it up.

In 1959, Hawaii became the fiftieth state. The Disney movie *Bambi* was released on that date in 1942. The Mona Lisa was stolen from the Louvre in 1911. It was recovered two years later, but it was because of this theft that the painting gained worldwide fame.

Famous birthdays include singer Kenny Rogers, basketball player Wilt Chamberlain, athlete Usain Bolt, gangster Bugs Moran, and comedian Bo Burnham. *SpongeBob SquarePants* creator Stephen Hillenburg was born on August 21, as was Joe Strummer of The Clash. My actual birthday is June 6, 1962. Only one thing ever happened on June 6 in the entire history of mankind: D-Day, the invasion of Normandy by Allied forces that began the end of World War II. I've seen every movie about D-day at least twenty times. *The Longest Day* had so many stars in it and is still one of the greatest movies ever made.

I know everything there is to know about D-day because it was somehow emphasized by everyone much more than my birthday. When I would ask people if they knew what day it was on June 6th, they'd reply, "D-day." I would always excitedly respond, "MY BIRTH-

DAY," in a loud voice, then storm off as if the universe itself were against me.

What I knew most about August 21 was that it was five days after Elvis died and it was the birthday of a close childhood friend. Nothing in particular stands out about the date, certainly no world-shaping event like D-day. If I walk up to strangers and ask if they know what day it is on August 21, all I get is a weird look, as if they're getting ready to call the police. I don't respond, "I died today," because then people think I'm really strange. (Well, I don't do that anymore.)

I don't approach August 21 with anxiety. I don't get depressed. I consider it a second birthday. I celebrate it. I embrace it. My family and I have a birthday party. I blow out candles on a cake like a little kid. Some friends call it my rebirthday. I receive congratulations and kind notes that day as if it were my regular birthday.

I celebrate in recognition of the two lives I lead: the one I had before I died, and the one I have now. It's an acceptance that I'm not the same person I was before. Close, but no cigar. It's okay, I have a wonderful life and plenty to look forward to. This is a much better way of approaching life than lamenting the person I'm never going to be, no matter how hard I try.

At the time of this writing, I am both fifty-nine and six years old.

Having two birthdays has its advantages. When someone tells me to act my age, I tell them that I'm six years old. I tell them I can't wait to turn eighteen so I can go to R-rated movies.

Treating my death anniversary as a day of celebration is easier for me than most survivors because I have almost zero recollection of my heart attack. I am fully aware of the pain surrounding it, such as wearing a life vest for a month with broken ribs. But I don't remember the pain of the event itself. I have heard from other trauma survivors who recall their event about how incredibly painful those moments were. If I'm being honest with myself, I'm grateful to have been spared that anxiety.

The question is: how can you turn your trauma anniversary from a day of dread into a day you can look forward to?

Other survivors have told me that they not only dread their

anniversary, but they spend days and even weeks feeling anxious as the date approaches. That sounds terrible!

I believe the best answer here is to turn something bad into something good. Spend your trauma anniversary doing something that makes you feel ALIVE. Spend the day with your grandchildren. Tell someone you love them. Go to a place that makes you feel at peace. Get up and watch the sun rise while you write in your gratitude journal.

One year, my family participated in a 5K dressed as superheroes, complete with masks and capes. I have photos of myself holding a giant number five balloon. It was silly, but effective. It helped put me in a celebratory mood to be outside, using my body, surrounded by those I love most.

Make a plan for your day and then stick to it. Go to breakfast at your favorite spot. Make love to your partner. Find something to make the day memorable for something more than your trauma. Not only will it distract you, but it will help you form a positive association with the day.

CHAPTER 18
ACCEPTING REALITY

UNFORTUNATELY, THERE ARE DAYS WHERE EVERYTHING GOES TO HELL. IT'S going to happen eventually. Maybe I have an awful night of sleep and feel terrible when I wake up in the morning. Maybe I become stressed about a problem at work that I can't solve. Maybe I have an argument with someone close to me and can't let it go.

Despite my best attempts to recover, fatigue overtakes me. Headache pain overwhelms me, and I find myself unable to think. I become nonfunctional. If it gets severe enough, I can't stand to look at any light, which means I can't even look at my phone as a distraction. That's when you know it's really bad: the one addiction we all share and I can't even take part.

In the past, I would try to power through my fatigue and headache pain. This is a terrible idea, as it only results in two bad days in a row instead of just one. I've finally realized that it's better to just write the day off and rest rather than push myself.

Losing an entire day like that is difficult because I pride myself on being a very productive person. I have many things I want to accomplish and wasting time doesn't fit into my agenda. I've mostly learned to forgive myself for wasted days, but I can sometimes get caught up in self-pity.

When that happens, I wish that my life would have ended. It's too difficult to go on, and no one would miss me. I see myself as a burden and just wish I was done. Society tells us that we're supposed to be constantly positive. It's a nice concept, but for many of us, it's completely unrealistic. The battle that some people fight daily is so difficult that we need to give ourselves a break from positivity once in a while. Even positivity can be toxic.

When I'm feeling like this, I need something that will drag me out of my malaise. It is then I remember Admiral James Stockdale and Stockdale's Paradox.

Jim Collins wrote the book, *Good to Great*, in which he interviewed Admiral Stockdale, a naval aviator who was taken prisoner during the Vietnam War. He was tortured throughout his captivity, which lasted from 1965 to 1971. Collins had read *In Love and War*, a book Stockdale and his wife had written about getting through his years as a POW. Collins stated that the book depressed him, even though he knew the ending: that Stockdale made it out alive and reunited with his family.

During the interview, Collins asked Stockdale how he held on and made it home:

If it feels depressing for me, how on earth did he deal with it when he was actually there and did not know the end of the story?

"I never lost faith in the end of the story," he said, when I asked him. "I never doubted not only that I would get out but also that I would prevail in the end and turn the experience into the defining event of my life, which, in retrospect, I would not trade."

Collins also asked Stockdale about the prisoners who didn't make it out of Vietnam:

"Oh, that's easy," he said. "The optimists."

"The optimists? I don't understand," I said, now completely confused, given what he'd said 100 meters earlier.

"The optimists? Oh, they were the ones who said, 'We're going to be out by Christmas,' and Christmas would come, and Christmas would go. Then they'd say, 'We're going to be out by Easter,' and Easter would come, and Easter would go. And then Thanksgiving, and then it would be Christmas again. And they died of a broken heart."

Stockdale then continued with a line that defined what Collins called Stockdale's Paradox:

"You must never confuse faith you will prevail in the end — which you can never afford to lose — with the discipline to confront the most brutal facts of your current reality, whatever they may be."

The brutal fact is that my life changed forever the day I died. No matter how hard I fight, no matter what I try, I will never be the same. I will live with the effects of that day forever. My brain is damaged. Part of my heart is dead. It took years for me to accept that I can't change that reality.

When the bad days come, I remember Stockdale's Paradox so I don't become disheartened about the future. If James Stockdale could endure years of torture and uncertainty, I can endure one bad day. I can make it to tomorrow, wake up, and start a new day with the hope that it will be better.

Stockdale's comment that he would turn his captivity into the defining event of his life and that he wouldn't trade it is noteworthy. I have told myself over and over that I wouldn't let my death define me, yet here I am, writing about it repeatedly. I have reclaimed much of my life. Others who have experienced extreme trauma haven't fared as well. I feel an obligation to tell others how I recovered, so perhaps they can too.

If a genie appeared, ready to grant me wishes, would I trade my death for a different kind of life? Only a madman would say no. My memories are shattered; how I would love to regain the memories of my children growing up. It would be heaven on earth if I didn't live with constant headache pain. I could do math again.

Unfortunately, the idea that I can change my life to that degree is a fantasy, and to pursue such a fantasy is folly. It only leads to more heartbreak. I can waste time hoping magic will happen or I can have new experiences and gain new memories to replace those that are gone. It's best to accept my death as a brutal fact and move on, so I don't waste any more time on the debate.

What does it mean to "prevail in the end?"

For me, it means to live a happy, fulfilled life. That sounds like a platitude, a statement you'd expect someone in public relations to say, even though it means nothing at all.

But to me, it means I stay true to my "Important List," and I stay healthy enough to travel with my wife. It means accomplishing goals, such as publishing this book to help people understand how to make it through the most difficult period of their lives. Before I'm done for good, I'd like to make it to Europe and publish a best-selling novel. I still have goals. I plan to meet them.

I find Stockdale's Paradox inspirational. It's not a Hallmark movie full of phony, feel-good fluff. It's about a person who went through hell and came out the other side damaged but better than before. That's what I want to do.

CHAPTER 19
QUESTIONS TO ASK YOUR CARDIOLOGIST

IT CAN BE OVERWHELMING TO MEET WITH YOUR CARDIOLOGIST AFTER YOUR heart attack. You're still reeling from the fact that you've had a major cardiac event, and it is normal to not be able to think of the important questions to ask on the spot. The questions here may or may not apply to your specific situation, since every heart attack and every survivor is different. These questions are a good place to start, a way to make the most of your time with your doctor. Write the answers down during the visit so you don't forget exactly what the doctor said.

Was my heart permanently damaged by my heart attack event?
Learning about the condition your heart is in will help you understand what you need to do to take care of it.

What is my EF?
EF stands for "ejection fraction." Ejection fraction is a measurement of the percentage of blood leaving your heart each time it contracts. It's basically a measurement of how well your heart works. A normal EF is between 50 and 70 percent.

. . .

What are my odds of having another heart attack, and what can I do to avoid one?

This question is standard for every heart attack survivor. If it doesn't come up in the doctor's office, it will come up late at night while you're trying to fall asleep. It will drive you crazy. Ask.

What are my medications and what do they do?

The better you understand your medication, the less likely you are to take something that may interact badly with them and cause a problem. This also means you are less likely to get anxious about them.

What if I miss a dose of my medication?

Not having the answer to this question plagued my wife and I with anxiety because I constantly forgot to take my pills. Knowing the answer ahead of time spares you the anxiety I experienced.

What can I take when I have a cold, the flu, or a stuffy nose?

We never seem to think of this until we're actually sick. Many over-the-counter medications can affect your blood pressure or interact with your existing medicine. It's best to know ahead of time.

What can I take when I can't sleep?

Some sleep aids may interact with your existing medication. Like cold medicine, it's best to consult with your doctor about what you should and should not take.

How much activity is okay for me? Will I be able to participate in sports (or other activities) as I did previously? How soon can I return to work?

We all have different levels of appropriate activity. Many heart attack survivors who were gym rats, runners, bicyclists, or outdoor enthusiasts will want to know if or when they can resume those activities.

Returning to work is an important step for almost everyone. Ask your doctor about what is safe, and you might also ask them what you should tell your employer. You may need a doctor's note to return to work.

What types of exercise are appropriate for me?

When I left the hospital, I was given recommendations on exercise. I was told to walk daily, and the amount increased each week. You may be given similar guidelines, but if you aren't, you should ask your doctor. It's important that you don't overexert yourself and end up back in the emergency room.

What causes my blood pressure to drop when I am on medication to regulate my blood pressure?

This was always confusing to me, and it would be nice to have an answer for it.

When do I take my nitro? (If prescribed)

I was prescribed nitroglycerine shortly after I was discharged. It's important to know what it does, how it will affect you, and when you should take it.

How important is a low-salt or no-salt diet?

I made the incorrect assumption that I needed to cut salt out of my diet. It would have saved me a lot of flavorless meals if I had consulted with my doctor first about salt intake.

· · ·

What changes in diet do I need to make?

Your doctor or cardiologist may have a specific diet they would like you to follow.

Do I need to make lifestyle changes? If so, what type?

There isn't a rational doctor alive who would advise you to keep smoking. They may also have recommendations on job-related stress, alcohol intake, or other factors that can influence your recovery.

Are periodic checkups necessary? How often?

I see my cardiologist at least once a year due to the severity of my heart attack.

Can I have sex?

It may be a while before you can return to sex, depending upon the severity of your heart attack. You may be eager to return to sexual intimacy, but it's better to be safe than sorry. Ask.

Is it safe to use Viagra or other medication for erectile dysfunction?

Taking Viagra concurrently with nitroglycerine can drop your blood pressure so low that it could kill you. Be aware of the side effects and get it cleared with your doctor.

How do I know when I need to call 911 or the local emergency number?

I like to avoid trips to the hospital at all costs, but I also don't want to ignore a serious problem. Knowing when you should call an emergency number versus when you can wait to see your regular doctor might spare you a lot of money and a huge amount of anxiety.

. . .

Should I measure my blood pressure regularly?

I never take my own blood pressure, but this might not be the right decision for everyone. Ask your doctor if it's necessary or helpful.

How long does it take an artery to clog before it becomes an issue for the heart?

Heart patients may have an artery blocked at 40 percent. It may not be an issue until it reaches a higher level, such as 70 percent. Ask your cardiologist about when it will become a problem and know the warning signs.

CHAPTER 20
RESOURCES

ADDRESSING THE STRUGGLES YOU WILL FACE AFTER A HEART ATTACK WILL be a very personal journey, and it is important to identify strategies that work for you. In this book, I have discussed the strategies that have helped me reclaim my life. They may not all be right for you, but they can be a great place to start. For additional resources and links to relevant articles and information, please visit my website at www.jon-johnston.com

PHYSICAL EXERCISE

Exercise is crucial to heart attack survivors. Before beginning any exercise regimen, consult your doctor to create a routine that is safe for your recovering heart. Be sure to understand your METs score; overexerting yourself can cause more damage and set you back in your recovery. Stop and rest if an activity causes pain or makes you dizzy or short of breath. Cardiac rehab is a great way to build up your stamina and get your body ready for regular exercise.

Insurance Provider

Many health insurance providers offer fitness incentives. Heidi earns points for staying fit and redeems them for Amazon gift cards.

She also earned a free Apple watch. Check with your provider to see if your plan offers this benefit.

Nike Training Club

This free mobile app offers workouts for every ability level, including yoga, HIT, core, and cardio. The NTC app can also be paired with an Apple watch.

Fitness Trackers

A fitness tracker is a great way to monitor your heart rate during exercise to avoid pushing yourself too hard. I love my Apple watch, but there are also many less expensive alternatives out there, including bands from Fitbit, Samsung, and Garmin. A heart rate monitor is a must, and if you swim regularly, look for waterproof models. Ask your doctor for target heart rate goals that are appropriate for you.

Getting Started

Any exercise plan should be approved by your doctor or rehabilitation therapist. Start small—begin by walking for a few minutes every day, and gradually add more time until you can comfortably exercise for thirty minutes. Here are some excellent heart-healthy exercises to get you started:

- Walking
- Jogging
- Swimming
- Biking
- Rowing
- Aerobics
- Yoga
- Dancing
- Gardening/Yard Work

MEDITATION/MINDFULNESS

In addition to the resources listed below, check with your local community center for classes or educational sessions, and visit YouTube for a wealth of videos on meditation.

Books

Mindfulness on the Go by Padraig O'Morain

Mindfulness on the Go by Jan Chozen Bays

Practicing Mindfulness by Matthew Sockolov

Self-Compassion: The Proven Power of Being Kind to Yourself by Kristin Neff

Wherever You Go, There You Are by Jon-Kabat-Zinn

The Miracle of Mindfulness: An Introduction to the Practice of Meditation by Thich Nhat Hanh

Apps

Calm – Perhaps the most well-known, featuring tons of guided meditation exercises and breathing techniques. Subscription required, but Calm offers a seven-day free trial.

Headspace – User-friendly interface offering hundreds of guided meditation exercises for both beginners and seasoned pros. Subscription required, but Headspace offers a two-week free trial.

Insight Timer – Free version offers thousands of meditation exercises. Premium version is relatively inexpensive, compared to Calm and Headspace.

Ten Percent Happier – Helps build a routine using streaks, and experts are available to answer your questions. Subscription required, but Ten Percent Happier offers a seven-day free trial.

Music

Music can be a great way to assist in your mindfulness practice and help you focus during work or difficult tasks. It takes trial and error to find the right type of music for you, so be patient!

Brain.fm – The best focus music I've found, but the app and website are clunky and in need of updating.

Spotify – So many options, including focus music, classical, and nature sounds. I enjoy a playlist called "Deep Focus."

YouTube – Another option for a wide variety of focus music and ambient sounds.

Headphones & Ear Plugs

Bose 700 – Over-ear, noise-canceling headphones with built-in microphone. Expensive, but excellent noise cancellation.

Bose QuietComfort 45 – Less expensive version of the 700.

Sony WH-1000XM4 – Less expensive than the Bose 700, but similar quality and noise cancellation.

Apple AirPods Max – Most expensive over-ear headphones on the list, but these pair beautifully with other Apple products and offer superb noise cancellation, spatial audio, and easy transparency mode.

Apple AirPods Pro – Earbuds with noise-canceling feature for less conspicuous noise control. They are very popular but didn't fit my ears well.

Powerbeats Pro Wireless Earbuds – Earbuds with an ear hook for people who are active. Less expensive than Apple AirPods and plays well with both Apple and Android devices.

Vibes Ear Plugs – Reduces sound levels by an average of 22dB while still allowing you to clearly hear those around you. Extremely discreet design.

Eargasm Ear Plugs – Slightly more expensive, similar performance, offers many options and sizes.

JOURNALING

All you really need to get started with journaling is a pencil and a piece of paper. The great thing about journaling is that it can be as simple or as fancy as you want to make it. For people like me who don't enjoy writing by hand, journaling apps offer a great alternative.

Day One – Beautiful, award-winning app that offers excellent privacy, the ability to add photos and videos, and voice transcription options. Available for the iPhone, Apple watch, and Mac. Unfortunately, Day One does not offer a Windows version. There is a free Basic version, but the Premium subscription is worth the cost.

Journey – Alternative to Day One that runs on Windows, Mac, Android, and iPhone. Subscription required.

Moodnotes – Great app for tracking mental health and well-being to identify triggers in your daily routine.

SLEEP: WEIGHTED BLANKETS

Weighted blankets provide "deep pressure stimulation," which can reduce anxiety and stress and encourage relaxation and sleep. Look for a blanket that is about 10% of your body weight (e.g., a person who weighs 150 pounds should look for a 15-pound blanket). This may require some experimentation, as some people prefer a slightly lighter or heavier blanket. Target and Amazon both offer many options, but most bedding retailers also carry weighted blankets.

Sleep Supplement

When I'm especially stressed, I use the "Sleep" supplement by Olly. It comes in gummy form, and contains melatonin, L-theanine, and botanicals.

HoMedics White Noise sound machine

Inexpensive device that plays white noise, thunder, ocean, rain, summer night, and brook sounds. Can play continuously or for 15, 30, or 60 minutes.

Dohm Classic sound machine

Some people are bothered by digitally produced sound, making the Dohm a great alternative. This fan-based sound machine offers two speed options and adjustable tone and volume.

MEMORY: NOTE-TAKING APPLICATIONS

I take a lot of notes, photos, and clippings of web articles. I sometimes copy clips or quotes from books. A variety of note-taking apps are available, so be sure to try several to find the one that works best for you. My favorites are Evernote, Microsoft OneNote, and Apple Notes. They all provide a sort of digital filing cabinet, a place to store photos, clips, and text and share them across your devices.

Reminder & To-Do Applications

I rely heavily on reminders and a digital calendar. Finding an app you love for your smart phone will give you access to your information on the go.

ToDoist – Extremely capable task manager for your To-Do list. Runs on every platform and offers free and subscription models.

Any.Do – Similar to ToDoist, this productivity app helps you stay organized. Easily share a grocery list, keep a digital calendar, and make notes in the daily planner. Runs on every platform and offers free and subscription models.

ACKNOWLEDGMENTS

Many people helped me complete this book, and for that, I am forever grateful.

Thank you to Tiffany Jayne Smith, Kerri DeLuca, and Vanessa Robbin for your invaluable feedback on the earliest draft of the book.

Thank you to Katie Lowery, my developmental and copy editor, without whom this book wouldn't be as polished as it is. I appreciate your willingness to point out when I'm being too sarcastic and not coming across as the decent person I want to be.

Thanks to Dr. Lou Kohl, my cardiologist, and Dr. David Willey, my family doctor for the past few decades, for your encouragement to write a book from the perspective of a survivor.

As always, my biggest thanks to my wife, Heidi, and our kids, Noah, Natalya, and Isaiah, for helping me heal. My life wouldn't be what it is without the four of you.

FROM THE AUTHOR

Having a heart attack is a lot like buying a car; you don't notice the model you're buying until after you've bought one, then you see the same car at every stoplight. You realize it's not unique, it's just one of many cars on the street.

When I started opening up to people about having a heart attack, others started opening themselves up to me. People from every part of my life began to tell me about their own heart issues or about their loved ones who were struggling with the same concerns.

Our circumstances were all different, but the outcome was largely the same: their healthcare providers had done a decent job of fixing the physical damage, but after leaving the hospital, they found themselves overwhelmed with emotion.

I wrote this book with them in mind. My memoir, *Been Dead, Never Been To Europe*, is a detailed account of my heart attack and recovery, but I didn't cover the specific problems I encountered nor did I discuss the strategies I used to recover.

If you're reading this, I assume you've endured trauma of your own. We spend a lot of time talking about "haters," those who bring negativity into our lives because it can be easier than bringing love. If we wish to live in a loving, compassionate world, love must be nurtured. I hope this book helps. I pray the best for you, and I send you my love.

––––––

Jon Johnston is an IT consultant and author currently living in Chaska, Minnesota with his wife Heidi, horse-dog Esther, and cat Leo. He is a native Nebraskan and therefore has an unhealthy obsession with college football. He is a heart attack and traumatic brain injury survivor.

If you'd like to stay in touch, please visit my website and sign up for my newsletter, **Jon's Postlife Crisis**:

Website: jonjohnston.com

Email: jj@jonjohnston.com

Precariously Perched Publishing

110139 Stanford Circle

Chaska, MN 55318

ISBN: 978-1-7358880-4-0

Printed in Great Britain
by Amazon

39495541R00067